Candle *in the* Night

Four Seasons in the Life of a Man with AIDS

by DUNCAN CAMPBELL

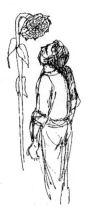

North Star Editions
1996

Text and cover design by Sara Glaser
Line drawings by Lee Weisman

ISBN: 0-916147-95-9

North Star Editions/Regent Press
For correspondence:
2447 Prince Street
Berkeley, CA 94705

Regent Press
6020-A Adeline
Oakland, CA 94608

First Printing, 1995
Printed on recycled paper

*A portion of the proceeds of this book
will go to the Hospice of Petaluma*

I dedicate this book to all refugees who have been turned back at the border, unable to land—refugees from war-torn countries and refugees from dysfunctional societies.

May you be happy. May you find peace.
May you be free from suffering.
May you find home.

Table of Contents

Acknowledgements

I am indebted to a number of friends for their help in making this book a reality:

For proofreading, I wish to thank Jeanne Pimentel, Victor Perera and Theresa Moraga.

Neil Herring and Lee Weisman took portions of the raw, handwritten manuscript and converted them into computer text.

Sara Glaser has done a beautiful job designing the book and book cover.

Lee Weisman has evoked several pieces in the book through her beautiful and sensitive drawings.

I am deeply grateful to Conrad Martel, my partner, for his patience with my passionate involvement with the writing. He has encouraged me along the way.

I hardly know how to thank my good friend and collaborator, Carolyn North, who took over more and more of the responsibilities as I became weaker. She has edited and re-edited the manuscript numerous times. When I could join her, we spent many a happy afternoon working together. From the very beginning, Carolyn has looked over my shoulder, offering excellent advice and encouragement.

And to all the friends who read portions of the manuscript at various stages, and who responded warmly, my deepest gratitude.

Introduction

I have been HIV positive for over ten years now. Since January 1994, I have been diagnosed with AIDS. Spiritually, it has been a turn of events that has intrigued me considerably. Initially I was terrified by the spectre of death I was facing. But through it all, I have welcomed the virus and the pilgrimage I knew it would take me on.

The place where life and death intersect has always fascinated me. Perhaps it's because I'm a Scorpio, sign of death and transformation. Fall and Spring are my favorite seasons when the potent mix of death and life is so rich, and the days are alive with energy and portent. The air is unusually sweet and musty, and the evening light is nothing short of mystical. I tingle with anticipation as each new day unfolds. I practically live outside.

I grew up in Oregon, where the land was verdant with trees and flowers. Even as a child I found beauty in brown shrivelled bracken as well as in lush green. Nature was abundant with astonishing treasures. To hold a cat's skull was to hold a prize at once awesome and sacred. It contained a mystery I somehow understood and was strongly drawn into, but could never have articulated. This is still pretty much true.

I entered upon the writing of this book with the naive perspective that life and death are separate entities. When you are alive, you live. When you die, you're dead. Simple. Neat. Through the process of paying closer attention to what is really going on, in talking with others, in uncovering some of my own motivations and aversions, I have come to see that life and death dance together constantly, the one lending meaning and context to the other. There is always the new and the falling away, always the rich composting and renewal. Always the intertwining of one with the other.

There are no points of arrival, only the process of transformation. The falling leaves and declined growth of summer represent a kind of death, a passing away. But in the truest sense, there is no death, no loss of energy. Only transmutation to new forms. The fallen leaves, twigs and branches make a thick mulch of dark humus that by Spring is alive with worms and their castings, a fertile layer of new soil. There is an awesome preparation of each season by the one that precedes it. Summer's lush growth collapses into Fall, providing the ingredients for the rich and secret alchemy of Winter. By Spring, the alchemist has provided the dark, living medium out of which new green explodes. It is a perfect run around a timeless track. Each season passes the baton to the next, and then drops back.

The major cycles of the heart often parallel the cycles of the year. As I learn to listen to the messages constantly offered by my body and my psyche, I come into closer alignment with the greater cycles of which we are all a part. The more time I spend in nature, the deeper and sweeter my connection to the seasons, both inner and outer.

I have written this book for you and also for myself. It is ultimately a personal journal in which I can trace my own process and discover my own path as it unfolds before me. It is a personal journal meant to be shared.

I have wanted to share my experiences, at least with family and friends, of living with AIDS, and to chronicle the shifts and evolution of my physical, emotional and spiritual states through the four seasons of this first year of disability. I wanted to leave something tangible behind that friends and family could hold after I am gone. I wrote this book so that I would be remembered, at least for a time.

It is a huge and awesome adventure, this moving slowly, inexorably into the final and full embrace of death. It is an adventure that excites me deeply, deserves my attention, is something, I think, worth communicating. It is a journey we all must engage in, sooner or later. If what I have written helps another human being struggling with illness, or with the ambivalence of living on in such a difficult age to have courage and a clearer perspective, to hear their own voice in mine, I will be thrilled to have made a positive difference in the world, to have strengthened the web.

Thank you for picking up this book. May its contents bless you.

Duncan Campbell
Laughing Crow Bungalow
Petaluma, California
July 4, 1995

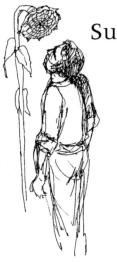

Summer

Diagnosis

MY HANDS ARE GRIPPING the edge of the counter of the pharmacy at Long's Drug Store, waiting for the prescriptions to be filled that will allow me to treat the Pneumocystis Carnii Pneumonia at home rather than in the hospital. Perspiration is pouring off my face and body. I have been running a temperature of 104 degrees for hours.

Less than an hour ago at the Early Intervention Clinic in Santa Rosa, Susan, the nurse practitioner, received the definitive test results of a long afternoon of testing. It was then that we knew for sure it was PCP. I had driven myself the half-hour north from Petaluma to the clinic, for a two o'clock appointment followed by chest X-rays and lab work at the Community Hospital a few miles away. I waited for the test results and finally reconvened with Susan. It is now 7:00 PM and I am on the last leg of a very long day. I can barely stand. My legs are shaking. My mind is nearly numb. I'm not going to last much longer before I collapse. I have not yet learned to ask for help when I am this weak. I am still used to driving myself, making my own decisions, and feeling a certain control over my life. But right now control and independence are the furthest things from my mind. I just hope I can hold out until I am safe at home in bed.

Finally a diagnosis! I am relieved. I suspected a month ago that I was developing pneumonia—the dry cough, the fevers, the terrible fatigue that made it nearly impossible to work, the strong desire to stop and rest. Finally in this past week, I had no choice. There was simply no energy left. I spent my time in bed. So I was convinced, but the tests had not yet detected it. Only today did the chest X-ray come back positive. Finally, the other shoe has dropped.

I was diagnosed HIV positive in 1986 and strongly suspect I was infected sometime between 1983 and 1985. A T-4 cell count of 160 brought with it an AIDS diagnosis in January of 1994. I was not surprised. I had been preparing for this diagnosis for nearly ten years. The progression of my illness was following a typical HIV positive pattern: ten years or more of good health and then a rapid decline.

I was relieved to finally have the diagnosis. Now I had a good excuse to stop working and go "into retirement," as we like to call it. I had not been able to say "no" to a huge garden project in Berkeley that felt like it was killing me. But I had made a promise over two years before. The original garden swept down the hillside in back of the French professor's house, full of perennial color cascading over stone wall terracing I had built. The garden opened out on a glorious panoramic view of the San Francisco Bay. It is a magnificent location and was my favorite garden. I used to spend long hours gardening there, immersed in the therapy of all that beautiful color, mostly blue, yellow and white with occasional bright splashes of orange and magenta.

Then the house and garden burned in the Oakland Hills fire of October 1991, leaving a scarred and blackened hillside. Neighbors and architects argued for a wide open view of the fabulous panorama. It was assumed by both the owner and myself that I would rebuild the garden to its old glory as soon as his house was replaced. But the old glory had depended heavily on a magnificent stand of eucalyptus trees at the bottom of the garden, and a tall redwood tree that together had framed the bay so beautifully, creating a noble container for the more ephemeral perennials. The perennials drew the attention, but the trees made it work. Even though the trees would have recovered, it was already determined by neighbors and the architect to get rid of the old beauties in favor of a wide-open panorama of the bay. So I was trying to design a garden for a large piece of property without trees that would grow taller than fifteen feet. I finally created groves of smaller trees but I was never happy with the results.

I started redesigning the garden with its new relationship to the house, not suspecting how stressful the project would be. Usually, I work in quiet seclusion at the back of a client's house. In this case, other houses were under noisy construction with radios blaring and the macho kind of energy I have managed to avoid most of my life. There were construction workers everywhere. Parking was a nightmare.

The old house had been a humble bungalow. The new house was an attractive double-story cedar shake house. Now all the garden walls and paths had to be pushed further down the hill and the main wall became grandly curved, where it had previously been simple and straight. Questions about elevations began to arise in the mind of the architect, and how the garden related to the new house. I had never worked with architects and contractors before; I was probably the only non-supervised non-contractor working in the neighborhood, and only once actually met with both architect and contractor.

The architect barely communicated with me at all, and when tons of sub-soil were dumped in the garden, the contractor only said, "Gee, sorry, but I didn't know. My boss never told me." The boss, of course, had disappeared to other jobs and the contractor couldn't be bothered. It was maddening. I soon found I was burned out as a designer; the ideas simply had dried up. I came to dread the drive from Petaluma and left more and more to my assistants. This lack of inspiration coupled with the severe fatigue of the last few months, left me depleted. But I persevered until I got sick.

Now, finally, I can stop!

The prescriptions are filled and I am home in bed with the breeze gently flapping against the curtains. I am relieved. I have nothing more to do than to sleep for as long as I want.

First Night

I WAS AWAKE when Conrad came to bed, having just changed the pads and towels I had soaked through with these persistent night sweats. We got to joking about the possible drug side effects they don't warn you about, and how refreshing it would be to see a list that went something like this: diarrhea, bone-marrow depletion, mental changes, bleeding, bruising, nausea, stomach upset, pale skin, fever, headache, blurred vision, ringing in ears, sore throat, dizziness, tingling of the hands or feet, increased appetite, loss of appetite, nervousness (so who wouldn't be, by this point?), mental changes, financial ruin, divorce, suicide, IRS audit, forgetting to water the garden, not understanding why the cat won't eat dinner on the same plate she just cleaned up after your partner fed her five minutes ago, death, extreme creativity, joy, dread, you name it—we got it. (Is there a renewed will to live in there anywhere?)

We're giddy. Conrad tells me Julie's joke:

Q. Why did Adam wear a fig leaf?

A. Because the man always wears the plants in the family.

I laugh hilariously, which catapults me into a major coughing jag, dissolving into my first tears in weeks, then sobs as Conrad moves over to hold me. "Hard, huh?" he whispers in my ear. I nod my head against his chest.

"I'm not sure why I'm crying—maybe some stored up tension ?" I remark finally. Again, we both burst out laughing at the obviousness of it. After things quiet down, we snuggle in closer, our hands finding the shoulders and cheeks (all eight of them) and hair they want to touch while our eyes gaze steadily into each other's and our faces mostly smile in a "how did I get so lucky?" kind of way. As we gaze, our eyes fall sad.

"Are you ready for the lights out?"

"Yeh."

"O.K."

Lights out, we spoon, the most delicious part of all. We crane our necks for the day's final kiss. "Good night, honey."

"Good night. Sleep well."

Its been a long day, and I'm grateful to be ending it with the man I love.

Next Day

SUSAN CALLS TO SEE HOW I AM DOING. She is delighted that the fever has gone down and says it is certainly not what she expected. She discourages me from watering the garden—even though I explain it only involves ten minutes of walking around with the hose. "Remember," she reminds me, "your other choice was the hospital. So be careful."

I put on my hat, go outside, and water the garden. Among the coreopsis and feverfew, the strongest of the iris are starting to bloom. Sky blue, old fashioned purple, white, bronze and midnight burgundy—the fragrances of my childhood greet me in each bloom. They are still settling in after the recent rude upheaval and replanting in their new home. It was a task that took nine of us to accomplish. Thank God for good friends.

We moved into this house April 1, 1994. I remember thinking during the two weeks it took to accomplish it, "This could be the job that kills me."

Yes, I see the possible connection with now having PCP I was definitely over my limits, both at work and with the move. But I have no regrets about the move. We played our cards extremely well, and to the best of our abilities. And look at where we are now. In our own home!

I no longer resent those last fifty iris plants I thought just might do me in. Nor do I think it strange to want to save every last one of their lives, although perhaps it is a bit ludicrous to have put their welfare before my own. But what's done is done. Now we are established in our own environment and I like it, this wonderful old Italian working-class house, solid, well-designed, generous kitchen, lots of light. Tony, who was a contractor, built the place in 1951 for himself and his wife, Lily. He died about eight years ago, and she, just a few months ago. We are the second owners. Their energy is everywhere in evidence: the fig tree next to the garage followed by the plum, pear and walnut. Then the spacious back garden, trees continuing along the property line: willow, red-leaf plum and a giant cottonwood. I love to sit under its branches in the Adirondack rocking chair. This is a place to be happy in.

4 P.M.: Down for a nap. I think we may be having a little drug reaction here. Amazing hallucinations, all changing with staggering rapidity, the images brilliant, beautiful. If I could capture even a single frame on film, I'd be famous. There are dragons in the curtains, very playful, following the sensuous lines, slithering past each other and disappearing in the folds, only to re-emerge in a ruffle. Friendly dragons. Time to sleep.

Quiet Mornings on the River

THE RIVER IS VERY PEACEFUL ON MONDAY MORNINGS. The crowds from the weekend have all gone. The old paddle wheeler, The Petaluma Queen, is docked in regal quietude in the alcove of water that serves as her berth across from this dock-side cafe. The loud calliope that dominates the area on the weekends is finally still.

It's going to be a hot summer. Today is a sample. Luxuriously warm. The few patrons at the Apple Box are clustered inside out of the heat, or under umbrellas at the tables scattered generously about the old timbered pier. Conversations are muted. Several of us sit individually at single tables at discreet intervals from one another, reading or watching or listening to stray words that reach us from those who sit together.

"She didn't!" "Really?" "all summer" "the boys" "In Umbria" "I loved it" "I should never have told him" "I'm so sorry" "You're kidding!" "How dreadful!" "It was on sale" "Tomorrow then…"

Actually, it is misleading to record these bits of overheard conversation in a string, side by side like beads in a necklace. There are long pauses of silence that intervene, in fact, the words more like a handful of beads broken from the string and spilled on the timbers one at a time, rolling away in random directions to lodge in cracks or fall through to the lapping water below. Very few discernible words escape the hushed conversations. The still morning air delivers truncated, intriguing coded messages to our little outposts of humanity at the furthest flung tables.

The old clock tower breaks the stillness, tolling the hour. Twelve o'clock. The tower breasts the horizon, as do more distant palm trees that must already have been adolescents when my grandmother lived here in the Twenties. I suppose the Petaluma Queen was really getting a grand old workout in those days.

High noon. I can hardly believe it. This place is crawling with activity most days at this hour, the old brick and stone walls by the river providing a colorful backdrop for the bright buzz of tourists and locals. The tin walls of the old mill gleam in the sun. Pigeons peck and fly in great communal circles, and then return to perching and preening.

Pleasant little chirps of baby sparrows bring me back to my own table. They hop about among the tables and chairs hoping for a handout, tiny beaks open and chirping.

The railroad track that runs past the tables is still in use, as I learned some weeks ago while David and I were sitting two strides away from it, totally unsuspecting. We looked up startled as a locomotive pulling two cars lumbered onto the groaning pier and rolled slowly past us to make its delivery to the granary two blocks away. It is a marvel that these old timbers, patched here and there with plywood boards, don't give way under all that weight. But there you have it. A train rolling right through the center of an outdoor cafe in downtown Petaluma.

Expect the unexpected.

Simple Pleasures

WE HAD OUR SECOND SESSION with Amanda, a therapist, this morning. I acknowledged that with a sense of normalcy and health returning, I am feeling a little bored. Now that I've come through the worst of my first illness I actually feel somewhat let down. I can still cling to Dr. Graziano's "three to six months to recover" if I feel the need to fend off would-be clients or others who might want a piece of my energy, but the truth is that with a little discretion over the weeks to come, I *feel* like I'm out of the woods and healthier and stronger than when I was first skirting them before going in.

"Why bored?" Amanda asks in her soft lilting way, tilting her head of cascading white hair. Outside her office window the redwoods descend to a little stream that has escaped the developers.

"Because the drama is over. The darkest part of the woods has now been explored and illuminated. I want to write and I'm running out of material. I feel like I need another illness in order to have something to say."

Both Amanda and Conrad are alarmed by this trend in my thinking.

"Why not write about what it's like to be healthy?" Conrad suggests. "Why isn't that valuable?"

"Because lots of people are healthy. What's to say? But if I can illuminate the experience of illness in a new way, then my writing may have some value for people."

But even as I say all of this, I know that Conrad is

right. I may not see as clearly what to write about when I'm feeling well, but maybe I'll discover what to say as I experience it and pay attention to its meanings and messages. Perhaps the non-dramatic moments spent in the Adirondack rocker under the cottonwood tree with its shifting patterns of light and shade are as important to record as the hallucinatory state induced by the latest drug I can't tolerate.

I suspect the sunflowers and cat may prove as central to my story of healing as the recent bout with pneumonia is central to my story of illness. Perhaps I will find that what we call "illness" is really just an aspect of a much larger process of coming into wholeness, into more complete health.

Life is unfolding in my own back yard. I'm not really *doing* anything, but what a gift it would be if I could pass along even a small fraction of the awe and wonder I feel watching the sunflowers thrust up through the zinnias and marigolds, or convey something of the sense of contentment I share with the cat when she curls up into a warm ball in my lap.

Simple pleasures. Profound gifts. These too are part of the journey into healing.

Sunflower

THESE SUNFLOWERS ASTONISH ME. I am a boy again. Jack and the beanstalk. Almost all of them are over six feet tall. How did they do that? It took me years to get this tall. They've accomplished it in exactly three months. In one third of the time it takes for a human baby to come into the light, they have grown from dry husks no bigger than my thumbnail, into giants already tracing the sun's daily progress across the sky with blind green heads on craning green necks. Their thick hairy stalks support heart-shaped leaves at regular intervals, some as small as my open hand while others are already the size of serving platters.

It was two weeks ago that the strongest and tallest arrested me one morning, head to head at our shared height of just over six feet. All my plans dissolved as I stood there rooted before it, captured by the potent energy emanating from the green head and its apparent consciousness. I felt suddenly apprehended, seen. It was like looking into a mirror at some essential green version of myself. Its yellow eye still tightly hidden, the powerful green presence was like an ancestor on the verge of speaking my name.

I have felt this with certain trees, their trunks mirroring my trunk, both the gnarled and the upright resonating in my deepest chambers. I have felt their full canopy of leaves call forth my own expansiveness of spirit, their stark winter form echo my own nakedness and strength.

I looked into the mirror and stepped through to the

other side. In that moment we both crossed over. There was no way to hide my brokenness from the green pervading my body. There was no defense against such strength and purity of being. I felt it inside me; my boundaries dissolved. Both friend and adversary, it seemed to know me better than I often know myself. It was like the rare friend of long years who, still charmed by your charm, cares enough to cut to where the spirit is both hiding from and hungering for the hard questions that only a true friend ever asks. Questions like: how are you really? Where does it hurt? What do you deeply care about? What are you doing with the rest of your life? Who are you really? What truly matters? What do you want? What do you need?

So what are your questions, my nonverbal friend? What are we asking of each other? Why does this sudden equality of height so stir my imagination? Why are you so provocative to me?

These are my questions upon gazing at you:

You stand apart from the others at the very front of the border. Why do you do that? Do you ever get lonely?

You are strong, upright, self-assured. Is it possible you are too independent, too proud?

All of your energy is dedicated to growing as fast and as tall as you can. How do you maintain such a clear focus, such strength of purpose?

Do you ever wish to forget your purpose and turn away from the sun? What are you giving up in order to be so tall, so clearly directed, so singularly focused? What would you lose if you let your gaze wander, if you let it follow the flash of scarlet at the fence as a hummingbird suddenly darts into the garden among the flowers, and as suddenly away? Does the raucous crow in the redwood tree or the buzz of bees or the swelling sea of marigolds and zinnias at your knees ever distract you from your upward thrust? Does the aimless white flitting of the butterflies ever cause you to pause? What would happen, I wonder, if you ever looked around?

These are my questions. I must live with them.

My life is growing quieter. Slowing down. Moving inward. I'm stepping back from the front row now, away from the front of the border and more deeply into the garden, into the shifting depths of light and shade. I seek the spotlight less often now, content to sing in a trio rather than up front as soloist. I've let go of the need to design a masterpiece garden, to compose, produce, and perform in my own shows—(and to get sick after every endeavor.)

There was a time for the spotlight; an important time. I had things that were mine, and mine alone to say. I needed to be witnessed, to be known by the crowd. I needed to know I could speak my truth and not be destroyed. I needed to claim my sense of belonging. I needed to find my place in the world.

Yes, I was sometimes lonely, sometimes proud, often terrified and needy, starved for applause. Those dynamics have not disappeared altogether, but the sense of urgency has finally subsided. I still need approval but I trust myself more, trust life more, trust people more. Perhaps it is a function of getting older, learning acceptance and compassion for myself and for others. Perhaps it's because I have done the work that was mine to do and have been rewarded with periods of genuine serenity. Perhaps the dragon has finally died. Just naming the demons has diminished their power. Wrestling with them is a soul saver.

I have walked through walls and passed through fire but always with someone holding my hand, holding the space in which I worked, casting a circle, making it sacred. I have hardly ever worked alone. I have always needed my teachers, my colleagues, friends. We journey together.

My demons would not let me rest. I tried to run away. They always pursued me. Finally, I learned to face them head on in the company of witnesses, many of them wise. We told our stories. We listened and learned. We cried when we needed to. We waited our turn. I thought the pressure would never let up, that the urgency would always pursue me. I am amazed to find myself resting, to be doing the work more peacefully now.

Perhaps it is because I finally valued myself enough that I was ready to live with someone as loving as Conrad, to learn what it takes to make a home, to feel secure in his affection, roll around in his humor, experience and learn from his strength and stability. He helps me believe. He holds me when I tremble. It is rare for me now to exhaust myself by running around constantly trying to please others. Home is finally a place to come home to.

And still it goes deeper, this place where I rest now that I've stepped back from the front of the border. I no longer try to name the unnameable, that which I grew up calling "God." But whatever it is, I trust it again and trust it more deeply. I've called it "The Water," "Great Spirit," "The Universe," "Caretaker." I've called it "The Mountain," "Great Mother," "Dear Father." I've called it the "Tao." But all of the names are too limiting. None of the names are true enough, big enough, silent enough. It's like trying to capture a butterfly by pinning it inside a box. Most of the time I simply say "thank you", without trying to name what is beyond my comprehension. But I believe it's there. It has shown me its hand. There are too many miracles and coincidences for me not to believe.

I am cautious about praying for things I want. If I pray at all it is to be aligned. I do not pray to be spared. I do not expect to be rescued from the path I am on. But more often now I trust that I am not alone as I take the next step.

Keep growing, sunflower, my green twin, my friend who provokes me with questions. I hope you'll open your yellow eye soon and take a look around.

There's so much to a garden, so much to see, to enjoy and contemplate, whether you're out there in front, as you are, my sunflower, or back here in the shade with me.

Flashing Yellow

I WAS IN THE GARDEN this morning on my way to cut a few zinnias for the house, when a tiny flash of yellow in the air caught my eye.

"One of the swallowtails," I thought with delight, glancing up into the blue air to find it. At the spot where I had seen the yellow flash, there, instead of a butterfly was my sunflower laughing in the breeze, winking at me for the first time from the yellow depths of its eye. Its lazy green lids were just barely drawn back like the unfolding petals of a camera shutter, or a sleepy cat's eye. The swelling green geometry of the past several weeks is coming undone, sepals yielding open to the yellow mystery within. I gazed up enchanted, just starting to focus on what I was seeing when suddenly the yellow disappeared again. For a split second I felt confused and abandoned. The moment I'd been yearning for these weeks was suddenly snatched away. Then I realized the breeze had caught up the green and turned the sunflower's head away. It bounced back winking and laughing at me, the sprightly yellow spirit peeking out from its green hiding place.

Laughing at me. Why does it feel like the universe is playing little jokes on me to get my attention? I haven't worked now for nearly two months, yet when I take time to sit still in the garden, the same message comes through that I've been hearing for several years.

"Slow down," it says in the most compassionate of

voices, murmuring through the cottonwood tree. "Slow down," the bees drone, moving from bloom to bloom under the hot sun. "Slow down," the white butterflies whisper, flitting in aimless, artless circles on their way through the garden.

I am amazed at how easily the days fill up: doctor, acupuncturist, nutritionist, therapist, case worker, lab technician, financial advisor, benefits counselor. There is weekly scheduling and monthly billing to keep the business alive and the maintenance crew going. There is mail to be answered and charities needing checks. Friends come to visit, and there's always the phone. Then there's the care of the garden (sweet garden): weeding and watering and cutting a few flowers. Some cooking, a little laundry. I feel like I'm barely doing my share. I sleep late mornings and nap afternoons. In the evenings it's support groups, rehearsals or relaxing with Conrad. These are not bad things. It is the life I have chosen, but it all goes so quickly. The days slip away. An anxious little voice asks, "Is this all there is? Am I doing enough? Am I living my life, or is it living me?"

The sunflower nods its teasing head.

"What are you saying 'yes' to? Are you answering my question or just toying with me?"

The sunflower keeps nodding, flashing its yellow eye like a...oh, I see! like a flashing yellow light!

"Warning. Slow down. Pay attention. You are coming to an intersection."

"Is that what you mean?" I ask the sunflower out loud.

Through the green leaves I hear laughter. The garden is alive with mischief. The sunflower keeps nodding. Flashing yellow. Flashing green.

Eye to Eye

THE TALLEST SUNFLOWER has finally reached its full height. I can barely reach the top set of leaves by standing on tip-toe with my feet in the grass. The yellow bloom of its eye is slowly opening. The actual head no longer follows the sun across the sky. It is bent over, as though staring at the spot in front of it where I stood arrested in wonder when first I realized how closely we're related. It seems to be waiting for me, holding my place. Perhaps it remembers our mystical merging, the penetrating sweet shock of mutual recognition as we stood head to head for the very first time. It waits for me at the front edge of the border, leaning forward a little on its thick hairy stalk, its huge heart-shaped leaves on strong stems like shoulders. Catching the sun. Casting shadows. Taller now, almost out of my reach. A master magician in a robe of shifting patterns of deep shade and sunlight conjuring up life from the ground, from the air.

These are exciting mornings. The air is delicious, fresh, alive. White butterflies flit among the unfolding brilliance of zinnias and marigolds. I come armed with my camera to record the daily progress of our back-yard miracle. So fast. So sure. So strong. Four days ago the yellow teased my eye, flashing and nodding from the green depths of the head. For another two days I've watched with wonder the elegant yellow fingers push out and split open the green gloves of the calyx, cells multiplying at a seemingly impossible rate.

This is the morning I have been waiting for. Today is the day I am certain it will open. This is the culmination of three and a half months of watching these intent green towers construct themselves in our garden. And now the tallest and strongest, *my* sunflower, has produced the very first bloom. I can hardly wait to bolt out of the house, past the garage under the shade of the fruit trees and into the sunny back garden to stand in the spot my friend holds for me, to look up into my mentor's perfect yellow face.

Yes! There it is! I see the flash of yellow as I round the corner of the garage. The flower is fully open, just as I expected. Exuberant in the morning breeze, it nods and dances, greeting me. Glorious yellow swimming in blue sky. The black crow loudly announces the event from the redwood tree next door for the benefit of the entire neighborhood. "The first sunflower is open! The first sunflower is open! Caw! Caw! Caw!"

I hurry across the garden filled with anticipation. The first thing I notice even before I reach my giant is the huge heart-shaped bib tucked under its chin, covered with a reckless spill of yellow pollen. I soon see the reason. Several honey bees are buzzing in ecstasy inside the finally-opened corolla. It seems I have not been the only one waiting for this event. One of them must have been working here since dawn. Her hind legs are bulging like saddle bags with yellow plunder and still she will not leave the bloom to unload the bags back at the ranch. She keeps adding more, using her other legs to stuff the saddlebags past the point of bursting. "Greedy beggar," I say to myself, smiling as more of the precious stuff spills down onto the leaf-bib.

The bees are captivating, an adventure in themselves, but my focus shifts back to the central character of my story—the sunflower itself. This is the great moment, the culmination of the life force thrusting up through the green, exploding into a joyous, golden mandala that shouts "Yes!" into the air with every fiber of its being. This is the miracle, the moment of truth. I am here to bear witness. The tallest and strongest has produced the perfect flower. My story of the sunflower is nearly complete.

But wait, what is this? My focus comes to rest on the very center of the flower. I feel my body stiffen, shifting in an instant from near bliss to outrage. There is an ugly gash through the very heart of my flower. Anger rises from my belly to my chest and up into my face. My eyes grow narrow, vicious with rage. My vision of perfection is laid waste, ruined. I see the culprit lurking, black body pressed hard against the back of the tunnel he's been creating in the secret darkness of the bud. No doubt sensing danger, he has gone very still. My finger shoots in angrily to pry him out, but to add to the insult, I am thwarted in my revenge. My finger is too large to reach him without ripping apart the tender florets on either side of his narrow trench. Incited, I reach into my pocket, refusing to be outdone by this loathsome creature. I whip out my comb and plunge it into the flower, along the offending tunnel and into the body of the earwig. Half of the body stays twitching in the flower while the other half comes away with my comb.

My chest is painfully clenched. I am sick with violence, and as suddenly, with remorse. This should not have happened. This was to be a story of perfection, but it has ended in a fiasco.

I thought to hide my shame at this outcome, and considered lying to project the ending I wanted—the blossoming of my perfect sunflower. Mine. In my garden. *My* happy ending.

But why? Why did the upward thrust of this giant

become a reflection of myself? And why did I select the most robust as my hero?

Perhaps it is because I am losing my heroes. So many friends failing, fallen. And myself in jeopardy, being bumped up ever closer to the front of the line. I wanted a model of perfect health to believe in, a refuge of my own where I could wrap those big, vibrant leaves around my body, hide in its stem, look out through its brilliant eye. I wanted to *be* the sunflower—the tallest, the strongest. I wanted the sunflower's energy as my own, an infusion of green, a new lease on life.

I love my body! I don't want to lose it!

My own violence shocks me, and makes me aware that I'm part of a much larger violence. The chronicles of the ongoing holocaust filter through and reach me, even though I avoid newspapers and their daily doses of despair. Everywhere the atrocities, the callous disregard for the sacredness of life.

Oh, sunflower, my sunflower, I cannot hold this pain. The grief is so deep, the need so great. I feel so small, so tired, so scared. I am implicated in crimes of commission, of silence, of violence, even in my own backyard. I need your forgiveness. I need my own.

I am only one, but I am one. I cannot do everything, but I can do something.

Am I doing enough? It will never be enough. But I am doing something. I am sitting here feeling, putting feelings into words, putting words onto paper, trying to tell a story. And trusting that the story may reach you somehow and elicit your own. Your story is essential. Do not be silent! We need each other's stories in order to stay alive.

Am I doing enough? It will never be enough. But I am doing something. I send checks to charities. I sing benefit concerts. I visit sick friends. I bring them flowers from the garden. Zinnias and marigolds, cosmos and roses. Sometimes I sing or read to them. Mostly I listen. Sometimes we nap or fall silent together.

I receive visitors who come to cheer me. This too is a gift, receiving others. We sit in the garden. We hear the leaves clapping over our heads. We talk about life and death and admire the sunflowers. We eat fresh figs. We laugh. We cry.

I trace the lines on my lover's face, from years of smiling, from recent pain. We leave each other love notes on the pillow, on the windshield of the truck. I laugh with him about simple things. I hold my lover and he holds me; with wonder, with passion, with care, with delight. Sometimes with sadness, anticipating loss.

I wrestle with my demons, and sometimes with angels. I try to show up. I try to tell the truth. I am committed to life for as long as I live.

Is it enough? It will never be enough. Am I enough? Oh yes, precious being, you have always been enough. Even when you didn't know yourself to be sacred, you have always been whole, you have always been enough.

I need your forgiveness, sunflower. I need my own.

Old Barn

THERE ARE TWO DIFFERENT WAYS to drive the twenty minutes north to my Monday night support group, by freeway or by back-country road. What a pleasure the discovery of the back roads has been! I'm still getting to know this county after moving from Berkeley two years ago. I've come to look forward to the drive there and back as much as the time with the group itself. Both experiences feed my spirit in ways I had not predicted. Both are of a piece for me—this treasure of my 'weekly adventure.'

Driving home tonight with the last of the sun streaming across the fields and painting the trunks of roadside Italian stonepines and eucalyptus to gold, I began to understand what it is about the back roads that so pleases me. Each time I come this way, I am surprised by something new that delights me with its age or perfect placement in the landscape. It is like opening a treasure chest again and again, each time to discover yet another jewel not seen before.

Today it was an old, untended walnut grove I'd not noticed before, the trees still robust even in neglect, a vibrant community of green on rugged black trunks between expansive fields of summer gold. Last week the perfectly square farmhouse seemed to step closer to the road as I passed. With no trees to hide its stark, weathered presence, its old white walls are visible for miles around. It seemed lonely and sad to me, but stood stalwart, its paint peeling straightforwardly without apology. The predictably spaced windows, as if blinded by constant exposure to the sun, appear to be looking inward, rather than out.

Cows, sheep, goats and old chicken coops are among my favorite sights, as are the miniature horses on one farm, and the field where llamas graze along with sheep, on another. Such surprises when first I saw them, they now are important old friends, bringing diversity and novelty to the landscape, as I myself do by my presence in a predominantly heterosexual community.

It is haying season, and today I passed field after field of golden stubble in which rectangular bales of hay lay at regular intervals, like big cubes of butter in the strong evening light. In one field, the baling machines had produced big tidy rolls rather than cubes, and the elongated purple shadows flowing from them across the gold palette of stubble brought Monet's studies of haystacks to mind.

An old barn with more boards missing than not, its roof entirely open to the sky, teeters on the brink of collapse—and yet has not collapsed. In the weeks I have been driving this route, I have come to trust that old barn to be there one more week, even another year. It is poignantly picturesque, moving me with its precariousness and inspiring me with its structural integrity. The barn's strong bones are still in place, bespeaking life well spent.

There is a woman in our support group who the doctors gave up on nearly ten years ago. They didn't take into account her iron will. Cardiomyopathy, diabetes, eighteen medications for the heart alone to keep her going, she's something of a phenomenon. She's a big Germanic woman with a grip in her hug as strong as any man's. The depth of integrity and expansiveness of her soul I have seldom, if ever, encountered before.

"I was so glad when you walked in," Martha told me, grasping both my hands after our first meeting. "Now *there's* an old soul, I said to myself." I felt flattered and deeply perceived all at once. My first real friend in Petaluma, Martha is a neighbor who lives just a few blocks away. I feel like I've known her forever. I believe her when she says we've had several past lives together. In the few short weeks I've known her, I have come to count on her being here every Monday, a landmark for me in the shifting landscape of illness and health surrounding us both. Like the old barn, she's solidly built and long-lived, with good bones and a strong will to persevere, and yet physically so vulnerable, so precarious.

Martha was not in group tonight. I must call her in the morning.

Martha's Not Well

I WAS RIGHT TO BE CONCERNED about Martha's absence yesterday. I visited her in the hospital today. She was admitted last night with a diabetic seizure and is being kept for observation because of her heart. Despite her robust frame, she looks very vulnerable in her flimsy hospital gown. She has a room to herself and was feeling bored, having forgotten to bring anything to read. I offered to sing for her.

"Oh, would you!" she exclaimed.

So I sang "Lullaby at Passage Time" to her, a song I composed during a time I spent pondering the dying process. Martha closed her eyes as I sang, and soon tears trickled down her cheeks.

Ancient trees hold up a sky thick with wheeling birds
Egrets nest while mallards muse among the reeds.
Timmy and I, as small as summer squash seeds
Float slowly on our tiny leaf-boats towards a rumored sea,
Dreaming of destinations we've never been before,
Zanzibar, Atlantis, the Moon.

And the water, the water, will lead us.
And the water, the water receives us.
Be a boat, be a light boat on the river,
Be the light, be the laughter in the water.

Emily comes drifting on a columbine,
Wordlessly conversing with her own mind.

Timmy slips from our leaf ship,
Humming themes from symphonies
While very gently alchemy
Is turning him to turquoise

And the water, the water will leads us,
And the water, the water receives us,
Be a boat, be a light boat on the river,
Be the light, be the laughter in the water.

Honeyed branches pass above beneath eternal blue.
Beaver builds while salmon swims towards history.
Evening comes gliding slowly toward the leaf boats
while turquoise changes into gold then indigo topaz.

And the water, the water will lead us,
And the water, the water receives us,
Be a boat, be a light boat on the river,
Be the light, be the laughter in the water.

We're drifting towards destinations we've never been before,
Zanzibar, Atlantis, the Moon.

Martha clasped both my hands, while we gazed into each others' eyes.

"That was so beautiful. Would you sing it at my memorial?"

"Yes," I replied. "I'd be honored to."

I left her long enough to get some books from home. I brought her my favorite ones—an old dog-eared copy of *Wind in the Willows* and May Sarton's *A Reckoning* and *As We Are Now*. She called later in the day to say she was loving *Wind in the Willows*.

"I'm glad," I told her. "I'll see you tomorrow."

Dementia

AFTER WEEKS OF HOT SUN and cool breezes conspiring to create a perfect summer, today is as grey as my mood. They say in group that we can always choose between love and fear. If it's really that simple, then I guess I've made my choice for now. I am resisting the urge to just go back to bed or to become engrossed in a good book to take my mind off what's really bothering me. My mind keeps returning to Bill.

Bill has dementia. I got the call last night.

I talked to his house-mate Bhavo and then to Bill himself who was in a lucid period. I agreed to take a regular turn sitting with him. Both his doctor and therapist concur that he can no longer be left alone. Bill said to me last night on the phone, "Honey, I want you to take away the ax when you come...and the cleavers. It scares me to have them here. I don't want to do a Lizzy Borden. I can't trust myself anymore."

"Sure Bill. Whatever you need."

The one thing I most fear about AIDS is happening to the friend with AIDS I most care about. I feel like the universe is laughing at me, pushing me in the direction I need to go next.

Bill and I met about six years ago in a choral group which sang AIDS benefit concerts in San Francisco and Berkeley. We were the strongest singers in the baritone section and contrived to sit next to each other. Somehow it became clear without our saying it that we were both infected with the HIV virus. He'd miss a rehearsal. I'd go blank in the middle of a line—that sort of thing. One night during a pause at rehearsal I asked him how he was doing. "I've been kind of low," he acknowledged. "I had to nap to get through the day." "Yeah, I know what you mean. I had to nap today too."

Bill is pretty private, but I felt he was letting me in more than before. After a pause, while we both pretended to be paying attention to the conductor, Bill turned to me and whispered, "Maybe one of these days we can take our naps together."

His dark eyes were full of mischief. It took me about two seconds to realize I was thrilled. I think I startled him when I whispered back,

"O.K., when ?"

So that was the beginning. We were week-end lovers for two years. I'd come across the Bay from Berkeley to see him in the city. We'd attend concerts together and occasionally get out of town for a weekend. We shared the same HIV status, and for an entire summer of weekends participated together in the STEPS program designed to empower people with AIDS. Bill is a long-term survivor, having been diagnosed with lymphadenopathy in 1981, already eight years before we met. Being very knowledge-able about the disease, he worked as administrative assistant for the Surveillance Division of the AIDS branch of the Public Health Department. Surveillance is the division that turns individual names into the death statistics necessary to chart trends in the epidemic and provide back-up data in the ongoing struggle for funding. Bill was both comfortable and invaluable in that job. It has been a sadness to him to have to give it up.

When we reached the two-year mark in our dating, Bill went into a bit of a panic. "What does this mean?" he asked me as we walked under the overhanging trees on his block in Cole Valley. "Are we in relationship? Are we lovers?" Given the fact that neither of us was dating anyone else, it seemed pretty clear to me. "I'd say so," I said. "Is that a problem for you?" Bill's eyes glazed over and he got very quiet. It was during that time I realized he had become sexually passive, and he acknowledged that sex seemed to be getting in the way of his spiritual practice. So we stopped being lovers and within three months I'd met Conrad.

Bill and I made the transition from lovers to friends with relative grace, saved in large part by our shared Symphony subscription, which brought me into town a couple of times a month. We'd go to dinner and catch up on each other's news, and then settle down into the red plush seats and just be together, arms and shoulders touching, feeling the other's comfortable presence as the music wafted up to us in the balcony at Davies Hall.

Bill's been sick several times since I've known him, and finally had to quit work sometime last year. He turned up in the hospital with severe dehydration and weight loss a few months ago. They kept him for a week of observation and sent him home only after insurance coverage became an issue. He fell once recently, face flat out on the sidewalk, because the neuropathy in his feet was so bad that his toe failed to communicate with his brain that it had tripped on a crack. The message did not reach his arms in time to break the fall. He's been under treatment for depression for months.

Three weeks ago Bill went into a psychotic episode that kept him sleepless and delusional for days. I wasn't there, but when I visited him a few days after the worst was over he kept asking me, "Am I making sense?" When I assured him that he was, he said, "Oh, but that's just on the surface. I'm good at that. You have no idea what's going on inside."

I held him close as we lay on his bed, running my hand over his short black hair, trying to calm his torrent of words, trying to encourage him to sleep. It was like petting the cat, waiting for her purring to start up, for her to relax and come into union.

"I'm so glad we've stayed friends," he said turning his head close to mine, his dark, dark eyes looming so close I couldn't focus and felt dizzy trying. Instinctively I pulled away so that I could really see him, but I could not hold his gaze, and grew nervous in the attempt. I quickly nuzzled my face against his neck and finally responded in a muffled voice,

"Me too, Billy. Me too."

My Grandmother's Blue Bowl

MY GRANDMOTHER'S BLUE BOWL sits on the low hand-carved altar she brought back from China. Most mornings I manage a little meditation. These days my ritual is kept pretty simple. After I let in the cat and we exchange our greetings, she winding herself about my legs as I open her food, I fill up grandmother's bowl with fresh water and set it back in the center of the table. Once or twice a week I cut fresh flowers from the garden to replace the ones that are aging. Then I take the square pillow from the window bench and set it down on the old Turkish prayer rug in front of the little altar carved with lotuses and Chinese characters I don't understand. I sit with my legs crossed and pick up the brass bells that hang on the leather thong connecting them. I strike them together.

It is the first clear voice of the morning.

I let them ring until the sound dies away, replace them on the bottom shelf of the bookcase and then light the candle that sits in a smaller, celadon-glazed bowl that a good friend gave me. I take the sage stick from its abalone shell and hold it over the flame until it glows red. I breathe in its sweet fragrance as I gently wave it in the air about my body. I dip my fingers in the water of my grandmother's bowl, bring them to my forehead and then to my heart. I murmur, "Thank you for today." My heart fills with gratitude, aware once more of the miracle that I am alive at all and housed in a body that still serves me well. Then I pick up the red book by Thich Nhat Hanh I've been reading, absorb a page or two, often the same pages I read the day before, letting the words sink in a little deeper.

All this takes about fifteen minutes. Finally, I fall silent to follow my breath and acknowledge the river of thoughts that float through my mind. Another fifteen minutes and I ring the little bells, blow out the candle, bow to my altar, slowly rise from the pillow and bow to it, too. The bowing keeps me from jumping into action. It slows me down, reminding me to reverence both beings and things as I go through my day. And I do it because it feels good in my body, like a very simple dance the Shakers might have done.

My grandmother's blue bowl is actually more green than blue. It is the blue-green you see in old turquoise rings in dusty antique shops in Santa Fe. "Robin-egg blue," my mother would call it. It is the color of the sea when it is boiling.

The bowl came from China along with the altar and many other *objets d'art* back in 1929, when my grandmother returned to the States after thirteen years of teaching there. She and her daughter—my mother—settled here in Petaluma up on Kentucky Street, not far from my acupuncturist's office. I remember the bowl years later in grandmother's hushed and refined University Women's Club apartment in Berkeley, after she had retired. I was a boy of eleven or twelve. It sat amongst her things on the carved rosewood shelves, in company with Quan Yin and Lao Tsiu, porcelain vases and exquisite rice bowls. It has always been my favorite piece; sculpted with fluted edges, reminiscent of camellias or petals of lotus. The rim is painted discretely gold. On the outside, exotic butterflies in elaborate colors hover in the white porcelain air. It is old and beautiful and contains many secrets. It reminds me of her.

This morning during my meditation my eyes focused on the water in my grandmother's bowl. The light was still dim coming in at the window and the flickering candle cast shadows upon the gilt rim. Images shifted in my head. The deep blue of Crater Lake. My grandmother sitting on the stone wall that rims the lake, smiling a rare smile out of an early color photograph taken on one of our frequent family outings. The image dissolves. Other images replace it. Camping trips with mom and dad and two older brothers during Oregon summers. The smell of pine from the hot canvas tent. The sizzle of bacon. The gentle clank of the Coleman stove. The call of morning birds. The slither of snakes. Hot sun diffused through pine boughs overhead. Underfoot, a carpet of needles fragrant in the heat. Lizards and stones, lichen and cones.

Return to the breath. Always return. I gaze into the dark depths of my grandmother's blue bowl, and like a recurring dream emerging from the swirling mists of sleep, floating up before me is the image of the snow crater.

I am twelve years old. Diamond Lake. My dad is the camp director, my mother the cook. Mount Theilson's jagged snow-capped peaks are perfectly mirrored in the blue lake water. Mount Bailey rises behind us through the woods. You can't see it from here, but you know that it's there, looming like a breast, gentle and forbidding. Its summit is the goal of the annual hike. I have been the camp mascot since the time I was four, tagging after my brothers and thirty other boys. Splashing in the lake and learning to swim, identifying wildflowers with my mother, chasing after butterflies, sitting around the campfire rubbing shoulders with the bigger boys while my dad tells awesome stories and night shadows dance and leap among the pines.

Sometimes I'd be allowed to go out in a boat with a

camp counselor, or one of my brothers. I remember the first time I saw the mountain. We had rowed out a little ways from the shore. I was intent on the privilege of handling the oars, my back toward the lake, facing in toward shore. The fir trees and pines ringing the lake gradually drifted away as the shoreline grew thin and the sky expanded above us. The squeak of the oarlocks and the inexpert splash of oars mingled with the lapping of waves against the side of the boat. The boat rocked gently. Elation and pride mixed with a deep peace inside me.

And then I saw it, rising high above the trees, a massive white curve filling up the sky. I caught my breath and held the dripping oars arrested above the water. Smooth and rounded like an overturned bowl in the camp kitchen, the mountain loomed. So unlike the jagged sharp peaks of Mount Theilson. Without thinking I took up the oars again, my unwavering focus steadfast on the mountain. It grew taller and broader as we got further out. It seemed so close, so terribly close. The distant trees were mere toys, like the green wiry pines on round wooden feet that were the landscape for our electric train set back home. Timberline was merely a green skirt in the near distance, above which the granite mountain rose up in earnest. Its upside-down image sought out the lake, filling up the blue both above and below. Across the choppy water it raced toward the boat. I pulled mightily on the oars. The mountain pursued us. Building up in my young body a wave of elation tinged with near terror crested and broke. My mouth flew open and released a long shriek as the image of the mountain finally overtook the boat.

The official camping age starts at thirteen. I'm only twelve but they've decided to make an exception for me. I am beside myself with excitement. I get to go on the annual hike! I have finally earned my right to be on the mountain with the men. They load me up with a forty-pound pack, a canteen of water, sunscreen and a hat. Mother steps forward and kisses me. I brush her away, hoping none of the boys have noticed. Finally, we're off. I adjust my pack. My new camera swings from its strap on my wrist. I am thrilled to be included with the older boys. I'm fond of Ted Hansen, the counselor bringing up the rear. He gently prods me along.

I have a tendency to drop behind, enchanted by trailside details and discoveries, in awe of the views opening all around me, wanting to take pictures of absolutely everything. I can't believe how fast the boys move. Aren't they looking at anything? There is so much to take in: the form of dead trees bleached and weathered by the wind, huge granite boulders rising up through the forest, the stunning view of Mount Theilson across the blue lake as the trees start thinning toward timberline. The lake itself, like a huge bowl below us. Enchanted and excited, I feel proud and powerful as I capture the image of the whole lake in my camera.

"I was here," I will say. "I saw this! and this! and this!"

I can hardly believe the majesty and power unfolding before me. Huge slopes of granite. Gnarly black pines. So much space! So much air! I am exhausting myself with sheer elation. I keep stopping Ted to show him this! and this! I am running out of film, and running out of steam. The pack is getting heavy, biting into my shoulders. I look up the trail and duty overtakes me. The sense of necessity to keep sight of the disappearing boys asserts itself into my consciousness and I try to catch up. I can't believe how fast they are going. I hear them laughing and calling up ahead. It seems like their voices are getting further away.

Ted is patient and indulgent, adjusting his pace to mine. He smiles at my outbursts of enthusiasm and only occasionally reminds me that we mustn't fall too far behind. Finally I settle into a dull plodding, one foot in front of the other, wanting desperately to sit down and rest. Up the mountain we creep into thinning air. Hawks circle in the sky, keeping track of our progress. The sun burns down hot, a fiery ball, unrelenting. The ground shimmers like horseflesh dislodging flies. A snake slithers across the path. Or was it a tree root? A lizard flicks its forked tongue at us, and is gone. The rock where he was sunning seems ominous in his absence. A cone crashes to the ground on the path just ahead.

My proud new boots are covered with red dust. They stumble over roots, collide painfully with stones. I need all of my attention to make the next step, and then the next, and again the next. My feet are burning, painful with blisters. My mind goes dull. I have forgotten Ted. I have forgotten everything but the tortuous task of keeping my feet moving one in front of the other. I hear in the distance the occasional call of the boys. I gauge my progress by the receding volume of their dream-like shouts. The voices no longer seem human, they are so far away. Perhaps it is the hawks shrieking high overhead, tiny black dots circling in the burning sky.

A root grabs at my boot and I nearly fall. The pack shifts painfully to one side, straps cutting sharply into my shoulders. I bring my glazed eyes back, startled into focus onto the wild path. The air is stifling, still, unbreathable. The trudge of my bootsteps is a heart beating in the dust.

If only I can make it to the dim outline of that tree up ahead. If only I can make it. If only...Everything I am is desperately concentrated, stripped bare, raw, essential.

Breathless as I reach and round the windswept carcass of the tree, I stumble dumbly to a dead halt, amazed. At my very feet it unfolds, unexpected, huge. A giant snow crater opening out beneath me. Scrubby pines vaguely ring the wide gaping rim. A cold wind howls up into my face from the yawning hole in the earth. My eyes drift down, down into the bowl and I catch sight of the boys far below, shrieking and sliding down the sides on the seats of their pants. I long to be part of them, but I know now with certain bitterness that I never will be. Their laughing presence on the mountain is a desecration to me. How can they raise their rough voices in an awesome place like this? How can they shout and sport and have fun?

The surrounding silence roars like wind in my ears. Far at the very bottom glisten turquoise blue pools—not one, but several in a field of ice. It is a color I never imagined existed, impossibly beautiful, untouchable, rare. Almost the color of my grandmother's favorite earrings, the aqua marines which she passed on to my mother, the ones I tell her make her eyes beautiful. But this blue is lighter, almost powder-blue, and yet deeper too, inaccessibly deep, rooted in the very bowels of the earth, impossibly beautiful, impossibly distant...

I feel myself fainting, my legs starting to buckle beneath me. I have been caught so completely, so totally off-guard. My eyes are filling up with tears. It had been enough for me to be included with the others, that it had never occurred to me to ask our destination. "Up the mountain" was all I had needed to know. I never dreamed that such a stabbing surprise lay in waiting, hidden at the very top of the climb. My legs are collapsing, my poor feet throbbing. My body cannot hold me. I crumple into a heap at the very rim of the crater, sobs crashing up through me again and again and again.

Ted's arm descends around my shoulders. I had forgotten him, but I'm so grateful he is here. And embarrassed. He pulls me over gently to rest up against him sitting silently beside me, his long legs over the rim of the crater.

"It's...just...that...it's...so...beautiful," I manage to whisper in a stammer before the sobs take me over and won't let me go.

"I know," he says gently. "I know."

My ears are stunned with the drumming silence.

I look down at the boys. They seem insignificant, like ants in sugar. You could rub them between your thumb and forefinger and they would be gone.

Morning light is filling up my grandmother's blue bowl.

Return to the breath. Always return.

The Needle Man

I'VE JUST COME FROM MY ACUPUNCTURIST. He says my lung pulse is stronger and my tongue is firm and stable, indicating good overall health. I am recovering well from the pneumonia. It's the kidney pulse that's weak.

He has me lie on my stomach, and deftly inserts two needles on either side of my spine right over the kidneys. I wince slightly as the needles go in.

"These are strong points. That's all we'll do for now," he says stroking my arm. "I'll be back in a bit. Would you like music on?"

"Yes," I mumble through the head opening in the body work table. I concentrate on my breath, trying to be peaceful.

In a few minutes he returns, takes out the needles and directs me to turn over onto my back. There is a gentle smile on his lips and our eyes connect, as they often do. "I'm just going to focus on the kidneys today," he says, pushing up my pant legs. He hums as he inserts three needles in either foot, two in each calf, one in my solar plexus and two in each hand. I focus on breathing, trying to be exhaling with each needle. They make me nervous. In less than half a minute all the needles are in. I breathe normally again, soaking up his calm. He smiles down at me.

"What can I do to help the kidney energy myself?" I ask.

His enigmatic smile broadens a little. "Oh, meditate, go to the ocean, spend time in the woods, strengthen your connection with nature. The kidneys are about containment and building of the Chi. The kidneys are the root, where the energy of our larger, connected nature can collect, like in a reservoir. Our interpersonal connections out in the world are often draining. It's important to replenish. We need to spend time in nature to reconnect with the source. Meditation, Tai Chi, Qigong—they all strengthen our life energy so that we're less vulnerable to being depleted."

"Is there an emotion that ties in with the kidneys?" I ask.

"Fear. Fear and vulnerability are associated with the kidneys, just as grief is associated with the lungs. The kidneys are also about spirit," he smiles, swiftly turning the needles, and then leaving me to rest.

"Fear, grief and spirit," I lie there reflecting, "my faithful companions. Will I ever learn how to balance these energies, to live less in fear, more in the spirit? Is one lifetime possibly long enough to shed all the tears I carry inside? Will I ever learn to love myself just the way I am, even as I continue to grow and change? Will my heart ever open wide enough to hold the whole world with compassion, to be connected to its glory and suffering without feeling overwhelmed or plunging into despair?"

"What can I do?" I had asked this sweet man whose wisdom I trust.

"Spend more time in nature," he had responded.

So, a trip to the ocean. I like that idea. It's been a long time since I watched the waves, I muse to myself.

My mind slows down as I drift under the calming influence of the needles and the profound kindness of the needle man. In my mind's ear I hear the remembered crash and sigh of the ocean drawing me deeper to the edge of dreams.

McClure's Beach

"WILL YOU BE ALRIGHT COMING BACK UP?" Conrad asks me as we prepare for the half-mile descent towards the beach. I look down the trail, steeper than I had expected.

"I think so. If not I'll just have to stop and rest along the way."

I appreciate his concern. It's a great comfort that he looks out for me this way. But I've been feeling good, capable, strong. Occasionally my chest still feels tight, uncomfortably constricted, and sometimes there are quick shooting pains that let me know I'm still healing. I take a deep breath, intentionally expanding my lungs as my acupuncturist has suggested. I breathe through the discomfort and come out on the other side of the pain in a place of expansion where my inner vision clears. It's been nearly three months since the diagnosis. Three to six months for recovery, they told me.

It's cold as we sit in the open doors of the truck, pulling on our socks and long pants. It was sunny in Petaluma when we left an hour ago, but here on the windswept bluff at the tip of Point Reyes the fog cuts like little knives into my T-shirted chest. It is still early in the morning. There are only two other cars in the lot.

I slip on my cream-colored denim shirt from Land's End, button it up against the chill, and then pull on the dark green sweater Bill gave me as we sorted through his collection the day we labeled all his drawers.

"Would you like this one?" he had asked me, checking

the label for "extra large."

"Yes, I really would," I responded, glad to have something of his to hold onto after he's gone. I feel Bill's love and desire to protect me as the warm dark green slips over my chest, covering my place of vulnerability.

Conrad rounds the truck and drops a kiss onto my forehead, his luxurious hair cascading like a warm curtain around our faces. "Are you ready?" he asks.

The fog swirls around us as we drop down into the gorge. Everywhere is the evidence of declining summer. Brown bracken and spent cow parsley with exquisite flat panicles of ripe brown seed pods on tall rigid stems grace the side of the trail. The ruined gold architecture of bent, broken grasses mingles with stone crop and late wildflowers, brave patches of life and color still clinging to summer in the midst of the elaborate brown wreckage of fall. Everything is descending, being drawn down, bleeding back into the earth; Summer constructs collapsing into the rich compost of Fall, everything inexorably drawn back to the source.

Our descending footsteps crunch on the gravel as our simple conversation dwindles into silence. Sandstone rises steeply up and away on the right. On the left the land drops down more gently and through the loud tread of our shoes on the gravel the sound of a clear, small voice reaches me. I stop to listen as Conrad continues on ahead. As his footsteps recede, the sparkling voice of a trickling stream declares itself as our companion, shy and playful and hidden among its overgrowing green, tumbling down the sloping thighs of the land with us to the sea. Conrad has stopped to wait for me. He too is listening. The little voice sings its clear song with delight, ornamenting the simple melody with bright burbles and trills. It is the only sound in the landscape, a perfect counterpoint to the vivid stillness of morning, the delicate spaciousness of air and expanding heart.

As we stand listening, my ear gradually tunes to the song of another singer. It is the voice of the ocean, the drone and thunder of distant waves muffled and dulled by the intervening land. My blood stirs and comes suddenly alive to the remembered thrill and terror at the sound of approaching bagpipes and thundering drums just before the flash of tartans and ribbons bursts into view at the far end of a wild rough glen. The broad highland chest that was my grandfather's and now mine instinctively expands, swelling my lungs full. The thrill intensifies as my flaring nostrils flood with the sweet scent of the sea. Blood and salt air rush to embrace. I stand sniffing the air like a bloodhound about to howl.

My heart thunders on the shores of my soul. My lungs are filled with the breath of life. I am more than myself. I am alive with meaning, with history, with portent. I stand transfixed, sensing, remembering. My body and spirit merge and mix with body and spirit from other times. Bone cries out and stone responds. Past and future flood into each other. Waves coming in. Waves going out. Waves crashing, mingling, dissolving back into source, back into one.

It is a timeless, ancient, jubilant homecoming, this rushing of blood and sea to embrace. It is a homecoming stretching back through generations, through bears and wildcats, lizards and snakes, whales and dolphins, blowfish and starfish, plankton and slime, back through jungles hung thick with vines, through ferns and briars, stone crop and thistle, moss and lichen, cactus and sage. It is a homecoming that stretches up into air, through trees and birds, through mountains and snow, clouds and sky, stars and comets and planets whirling in silent space. It is a homecoming stretching down into the ground, through roots, through stone, down to the fire in the very belly of the earth.

And forward it stretches to embrace what will come, into an uncertain future still swirling with mist, with terror and hope, with mystery and awe, with strange children full of promise and struggle.

My pulse quickens. I'm ready to move. We too are descending, along with the stream, along with the bracken and broken reeds, following the path, being drawn down, being drawn back toward home. I catch up with Conrad and we touch without words, sparkling eyes, gentle smiles, a rubbing of shoulders. We are being softened, molded by the morning, the sweet air, the sound of the sea. The fog is stirring, gradually lifting, like veils being leisurely removed one by one. We drop down along the path, following the little stream. It too is casting off its veils, green garments slipping away and being left behind as the landscape gives way to sand and stone. Naked to the sea, no longer hiding, the little stream tumbles and dances and sings. Already in my mind I see it flowing out to meet the ocean, surrendering itself, being submerged and subsumed. We round a final bluff and there the sandy beach opens out before us, wide and gray, the full force of the ocean still muffled behind one last sandy rise. Seabirds are riding the morning air. The little stream lets go of its song and flows peacefully onto the expanse of sand where it spreads out into several channels and then disappears underground before ever reaching the sea. It is not what I expected. There is no joyful reunion, no watery embrace, no tumbling into each other's arms. The little stream simply and quietly disappears.

I am drawn by the sound of the waves. I want to move on over the rise. Conrad stops to play with the stream, a little boy delighted with dams and diversions. He's cutting a new channel for the water, blocking off the main flow with driftwood boards, seeing if he can extend the reach of the stream closer to the ocean before it dies in the sand. I watch his delight and find myself smiling.

I am reminded of how my mother irrigated our vegetable garden on hot summer days by blocking and opening little earth dams, sending the water spilling down the rows of beets, carrots, zucchini and chard, asparagus, rhubarb, strawberries and corn. I would watch the water surge into the new channel, the leading finger quickly exploring the terrain, flowing around dirt clods, chasing beetles, turning fallen stray leaves into boats. Then gradually the flow would slacken, the finger become sluggish as the water seeped into the soil of the mounded rows. Slowly, slowly, nearly spent, the trickle would finally reach the end of the row and with no place to go the water would gradually swell to fill up the ditch. Then mother would divert it to the next row. Water meant life for the garden and food for us.

The sea is calling me, insistent, impatient. Leaving Conrad to play with the stream, I eagerly walk the short distance up over the rise, hungry for the thundering waves. The booming intensifies with every step. I clear the sandy rise and the sound breaks upon me, sweeps through me, devours me utterly. I am giddy and sad, shaken and serene. Standing before the pounding waves I suddenly hear hundreds, thousands of Taiko drummers, see their naked bodies stretching left and right into the distance as far as the eye can see, thundering on the drums, thundering out life, thundering out the world, the sea, the air, thundering out breath, making my lungs swell, thundering raw energy into the land, into my body, into the very marrow of my bones. The magnificent bodies thunder on the drums with total commitment of body and soul, pledging every ounce of strength they possess to the sound of the drums, to the thunder, the terrible thunder of life.

I stand for a long time taking it in. Then out of the corner of my eye I see Conrad exploring the beach. I notice the gulls gliding silently overhead. I turn to follow him, padding behind like a contented puppy sniffing the air. We are loosely following the line of detritus the last high tide has flung onto the beach. Brown seaweed, broken shells, tangles of string, occasional plastic. Conrad doubles back to drop a beautiful little stone in my hand, perfectly smooth and sensuously rounded, black and white. "Granite?" I wonder. "Pretty," I say. Our eyes meet, happy, not needing words.

Up toward the cliffs an encampment of human drifters is stirring, hair disheveled, pulling on shirts, moving slowly, waking up to the day. The air is growing warmer through the last of the fog. Patches of blue are breaking through the swirling high mist.

I nearly step on a spiral shell, half eaten away to reveal its architecture. Like a staircase spiraling inside a tower in an Escher painting, going up, going down. I pick up the shell and hold it in my hand. My mind flashes on lizards turning into frogs, into birds, flying away.

A life was lived here inside this broken house. The old house is beautiful. The dissipation of time has only added to its beauty, worn away half the walls, revealing the strong lovely form of the interior. It is an exquisitely organized structure. I wonder at the creature that built such a home. Like the sunflowers in my garden, it must have known exactly what it was doing to have constructed with such singleness of purpose this perfection of form. The house is like an echo of a life well-lived, the outer structure brilliantly organized around an inner sense of order.

There's a message here for me in the spiral, in the broken house with its integrity and strength of design. How long ago, I wonder, did the creature who lived here leave its shell on the beach where a man struggling to come to terms with mortality would bend to retrieve it, taking it home to wonder about its message, wonder at its gift?

A gift from the sea. Anne Morrow Lindbergh. I smile with fond memory. I am not alone. I am neither the first nor last to receive a gift from the sea, to wrestle with its meanings. The land, the sea, the air, the fire all constantly present themselves to us. All we need do is take the time to see, to listen, to ponder.

I rush to show Conrad my latest treasure. He turns smiling to greet me holding a crab shell against his chest like a brooch. We are decorating ourselves with the sea. We walk together now, deliciously at one as I weave green sea grass into a bracelet, inserting white feathers and red tufts of seaweed like jewels.

Conrad has found a big, dying crab washed onto its back by the tide. Its pincers stumble back into life, weakly moving in remembered defense as Conrad picks it up from the sand. He hands it to me. I am startled by the lively weight of its body, so heavy still inside the shell. The weight of a life. But the swarm of sand fleas and sand flies have already begun their work. The eyes have been eaten away. I feel terribly sad, and chagrined too, aware that we have robbed a fellow creature of its last shred of dignity, intruded upon its right to die in privacy, undisturbed. Something sacred was going on here which we interrupted. I place the agitated crab back on the sand as gently as possible, on its back the way we had found it. A prayer with no words is locked inside my chest, feebly moving its claws, blindly trying to scuttle into the light.

Conrad moves ahead of me again down the beach. I

wonder if he needs to be alone with his grief, with his thoughts of his previous lover Larry, whose ashes he scattered here three years ago. I tag along behind, no longer content. There are things here bigger than I can grasp, things that exclude me, things that don't need me for their existence or demise.

For a moment I feel disconnected, alone.

But then Conrad turns to wait for me, having reached the end of the beach where the cliff rocks march out into the sea. I run to cover the distance between us.

"Where's Larry?" I ask, a little breathless as I reach him.

Conrad looks at me quizzically, perhaps caught up short by the bluntness of my question. He quickly recovers. "Oh, all over here by now," he responds, taking in the rocks, the beach, the sea and the horizon with the sweep of his hand. Behind him the rocks tower like an impenetrable wall, dark, almost black, casting shadows on the sand. We follow the wall along toward the sea and suddenly a cleft in the rock opens up like a doorway. Conrad steps though. He has been here before.

I scramble behind him over sea-tumbled stones into the sheltering embrace of a small cove. Conrad wanders on ahead out of sight around another outcropping of stone. I sink down against the dark wall onto the sand to take in this new environment. There are huge stone monoliths in the little bay breaking the force of the incoming ocean. The waves lap gently onto the beach almost like the waves of a lake. I settle into sitting, watching, musing.

Within minutes Conrad returns from around his corner and waves for me to come join him. I feel a little irritated and consider waving him away, but I also trust him and know he would not be disturbing me if it weren't for a good reason. I climb up into my body once more and shove away from the wall. As I reach where he is standing, he cautions me to silence and points out to sea. My eyes gradually adjust to the brown and black forms of the rocks. One of them moves and I suddenly discern the wary head of a sealion rising above its brown mountain of flesh. We three keep watch, one sealion, two men, our mutual gaze bridging the intervening distance of water, of time. It turns into a waiting game. The sealion wins, finally relaxing back into napping as we wander away to find other marvels.

"Would you like to come out on the point with me?" Conrad asks before I can settle back down against the wall. I'm feeling tired and want to rest. But out on the point, he's told me, is where they gathered to scatter Larry's ashes. This is a clear invitation to be included with Conrad and Larry. I feel honored and humble.

"Yes, I'll come."

We start the ascent up over the rocks. Has the light shifted or is it the geology? These rocks are almost blindingly white, somewhere between sandstone and chalk. There are hollows in the rock where seawater has been trapped and evaporated, leaving behind deposits of salt. I taste a pinch of the crystals. Oh yes, it's salt alright. Strong, elemental, waking the senses. I am pleased. The path is treacherous across loose scree. I remember bounding across similar landscapes as a boy, sure of my step, of my body's intimate connection with the land. Now I crawl like a crab, finding handholds in the larger rocks before shifting my feet.

I am aware of the swirling sea gaining distance below me. The sun must be out. The water is blue. My legs are growing shaky. I am reaching my limits. A false step could send me crashing into the sea. I crawl along carefully, wanting to cry. I feel myself being softened, surrendering to these strange bouts of weakness. I am being pulled down, slowly, inexorably. Someday I will fall from the face of the cliff. I am not a mountain goat. I am not the boy who bounded from rock to rock. I am a middle-aged man with a disease that is threatening to take my life.

I may need help to climb the rocks. I may be weary and vulnerable. But there are gifts in the path and companions on the journey. I am not alone. A strong man who loves me is just up ahead. If I call, he will turn and come back to me. Even if he were not here, I would not be alone. There are friends both living and gone. There are angels and guides. Broken shells and dying crabs are all helping me along my way. I feel myself being softened, molded by the land and the slow, shaky motion of my body upon it, by the dazzling light reflecting off the water below, by the sound of crashing waves and the nearness of my mate.

I make it finally to the place where he is sitting, at the edge of a sheer drop overlooking a blow hole. The sea explodes and recedes. I come to rest against his body. He takes my hand. All is well. We are surrounded by the sea. Almost within a stone's throw, a huge monolith rises up above the reach of the waves, capped with the white guano of seabirds, like a mountain in snow. A flock of pelicans circles and settles onto the summit. A pair of gulls flies directly overhead. Another wall of stone steeply descends into tidepools directly beneath us. A tidepool opens below like a giant jewel box, a full two feet of an extensive colony of jet-black mussels cleaving to the sides just above the churning water. Here and there against the black are scattered brilliant coral starfish, mostly bright orange, but some as red as bloody rubies. Every inch of the floor is packed with rare emeralds, a thriving colony of green anemone opening and closing with the waves.

"Over there we gathered in a circle to say good-bye to Larry." Conrad points back behind us to a broad slab of stone. I notice the salt deposits, the sheltering walls. It has the feel of a sacred gathering.

"The women were all here and his doctor, Tom Crane." They had taken care of Larry for over three years. "Shelly was here and Anne came from L.A." Shelly, his ex-wife. Anne, his daughter. "David stayed away. He never showed up through the entire illness." David, the lost son who never came home but called for the oak table after his father was gone.

"I scattered the ashes onto the rocks so that Larry could linger a little longer."

"I imagine the weather has washed them away by now," I muse looking out past the jagged rocks.

"Most of him would have been washed away with the winter, but some of him I'm sure is still here in the rocks, lodged in the crevices."

We turn our heads back silently, gazing down to the tide-pools crowded with life in the wash of the sea. All around us the mists are boiling. Behind us the sky is open and blue, lighting the stone slab and surrounding walls. Before us the last remnant of fog is a dark shroud swirling with unanswered questions. Waves coming in. Waves going out. Two men watching, or possibly three.

A black cormorant still dripping wet from the sea flies screaming into the shelter between the walls, rests for a moment on a rock above the mussels and with another piercing, haunting, long cry catapults out again into the wild spray.

I have shifted back a little way from the edge, still within touching distance of Conrad but no longer touching. I am watching him sitting in the midst of contradiction, light pouring in from behind, a black wall of stone and fog before him. Between the dark walls I see colors forming in the mist, very near to where he is sitting. "Look a rainbow!" I exclaim, pointing.

"A fogbow," Conrad responds with a smile.

"A halo, actually," I say to myself as the curve of color grows in the mist, perfectly framing his windblown hair.

"Let's go home," one of us says.

A handful of new people are on the beach as we step back through the magic gate in the wall, leaving the swirling mist behind. A man and a woman with two small children, a boy and a girl, explore the tideline, offering each other their just-found treasures. Further down the beach a lone man trails his feet slowly through the sand, hands behind his back, thoughtful, occasionally looking out toward the water. Two beautiful young women strip to bikinis, dash into the sea. The sun is hot. Conrad and I slip off our various sweaters and shirts and loosely tie them about our waists, ambling the rest of the way with bare chests.

When we reach the stream, there are two young men extending the channel Conrad created. "Continuing my work," he says with a mixture of pride and humor. We stop to chat and then head up the path. The little stream greets us with its glad, sparkling song like a good friend who has awaited our return. "Another homecoming," I muse. "No, not another. All one and the same."

In my pocket I am tracing the lines of the spiral, going up, going down, lizards and frogs turning into birds, taking flight. Spiraling, spiraling, circling out, circling up, ascending, descending, continuing to whirl, embracing all directions again and again, spiraling to a point, pointing toward the future, intimations of infinity. Infinite connections, transmutations, disintegrations, ever new constructions, energy continuing, creating new forms.

"Continuing my work." Yes, my beloved, your work, your play, your life is continued. Your love is not lost. The play goes on. Our lives extend out in countless directions. Lives overlapping, one picking up where another leaves off. I stood today on the same rocks on which you and Larry once stood together. Larry and I never met in this lifetime, but you are the living, loving bridge between us.

You and I will probably never see the young men again, the two young men extending the channel for the stream. They picked up the game we had left behind and with their attention they made it new. We may never see those two again, but for a moment we touched, our lives intersected, we recognized something of ourselves in each other. Some nourishing exchange of energy passed between us. Water was the game that drew us together. Life is the web that continues to connect us.

Waves flowing in, waves flowing out. Waves overlapping, embracing, letting go. Mingling, merging, flowing back to the source. Everything connected, constantly in motion, spiraling, spiraling, ever new, ever old. Everything continues. Everything changes. Nothing is lost. Nothing stays the same.

Names are treacherous. "Yours." "Mine."

Is it a lizard, a frog or a bird? Was I a fish, an eagle, a man? Are you my lover or a visiting angel?

They are only masks we take off and put on. We are more than ourselves, alive with connection and shimmering shared energy. We are vibrant with meaning, with history, with portent. Our names do not stop us. Our bodies do not confine us. We are part of a great web and the web is spiraling. Spiraling up, spiraling down, spiraling out in ever widening circles, spiraling in towards home.

The ascent is easy. Where did all of this energy come from? I squeeze the spiral shell in my pocket and take Conrad's warm hand in my own. We pull each other close for a kiss and continue up the ascending path hand in hand.

We continue until it is time to change. Change direction. Change our names.

Behind us the sound of thunder is growing dim. Waves crashing in. Waves flooding out. Waves intermingling, overlapping, merging. Waves embracing and letting go. Waves dissolving and melting again and again back into source, back into one.

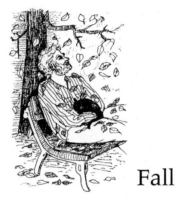

Fall

T-Cells

MY NEW DOCTOR AT KAISER called this morning with lab results. T-4 cells are down to 40 he said, down from 180 three months ago, down from 360 last year at this time. Normal range: 430–1,800.

"A significant decline." His words. Bill used to joke that when they dropped to ten I could start naming them!

The chest x-ray is clear, just as it was a month before I was diagnosed with Pneumocystis pneumonia. I'm coughing off and on, dry and nonproductive. My chest is tight. Is this unexpressed grief or undiagnosed pneumonia? Are the two related? Would a good cry relieve the symptoms, keep the pneumonia at bay? How are our emotions and will linked to our health? We know from the research of recent years that the mind and its attitudes do have a definite effect on health. Psychoimmunology is a newly developed field of medicine. To what extent would giving in to the desire for death hasten it towards me? Or if I clearly wanted to live and was giving my body that message, how much power would that have in slowing or stopping the progress of AIDS in my body? Old people in homes often pray to be released and yet they continue on for years while others clinging tenaciously to life are forced to let go. Whatever meaning there may be in such contradictions, it eludes me. My mind strains to understand, to gain some control, to find a perspective that can quiet the storm brewing in my heart.

Snowy Egret

IT FEELS LIKE I'VE BEEN DEPRESSED for weeks. It has been hard to believe it would ever go away. This morning I was so low, I actually thought about just giving up, stopping my medications and waiting for the next opportunistic infection to come along and kill me. Passive suicide. I felt miserable, body, mind and soul. I remembered no tools. I pulled on a T-shirt and jeans, slipped into my Birkenstocks and headed across town to keep an appointment with my acupuncturist.

In the little treatment room I sit disconsolate, staring at the charts and colored drawings of a naked Oriental man on the opposite wall. All over his body are tiny black dots connected by fine red lines, accompanied by Chinese characters naming each point. After a short while the door opens, and the little room is suddenly flooded with bright light from the hallway, casting a brilliant aura around my acupuncturist's shadowy figure. I am reminded of images I've seen on TV of purported near-death experiences where long-lost family members and friends step forward to greet the newly departed in a blindingly beautiful tunnel of streaming white light.

"Oh, it's you," he says, sounding startled as he enters the room and his eyes adjust to me sitting in the dim light. I am not surprised he doesn't recognize me right away. He has never before seen me with so little spark. I am slumped over, dressed carelessly, hair uncombed. Whatever energy I have is totally turned in on itself.

"How are you doing?" he asks with his usual concern as he pulls up a stool and looks searchingly into my eyes.

I blurt it all out, how my chest is painfully tight, how close to despair I feel, how little anything seems to be helping. How I feel increasingly like just giving up. As always, he listens very carefully. I feel his concern and compassion. He is taking me seriously. He is loving me, helping me to love myself a little. I am full of harsh self-judgment for not having shaken off this stupid depression with the help of the many spiritual tools at my disposal. His kind concern models for me a more compassionate response. Even in these first few minutes together, I feel the benefit of his calm, sweet presence. Something inside me begins to let go a little, his kindness making tears start up in my eyes. I am aware of how much I am holding, how much I have needed someone to understand.

"Why don't you lie down on the table and I'll check your pulses," he gently directs. On the table I lie in my tight, constricted body. He takes my pulses, three for each wrist. "Let me see your tongue." I oblige him, making the face of a gargoyle. "Hmm," he intones thoughtfully.

"How are the pulses?" I want to know.

"Cold and deep."

"Like death," I think, aware I'm being morbid.

He's concerned about the lungs and asks me to take off my shirt so he can listen with the stethoscope. "There's a little congestion in the lower left quadrant. I'll do the usual needles for the immune system and then I'd like to focus on the lungs."

"O.K." I respond in a dull monotone.

"I think you may have to slip off your jeans."

I know he has to get to the points on my legs. I know to wear loose pants when I come here, but today I didn't remember—or just didn't care.

"But I didn't wear underpants." I feel stupid and vulnerable. I always wear underwear when I go to the acupuncturist.

"I don't mind," he says reasonably.

"But I do!" I mutter to myself. I wrestle the pant legs up to my knees, rehearsing the unwelcome image of lying without them, still and exposed. "Like a cadaver," I think.

"Will that do?" I ask him, finishing my little task.

"That's fine."

Never have I responded to the needles so strongly. Oh, it's true that sometimes there's a little prick of pain. But not like this. As he inserts the first needle into my left calf, I let out a loud yelp, my leg pulling violently away from the pain. I burst into loud tears, trying to stifle them, aware of the thin walls between me and the patient in the next room.

"I'm sorry," he says, as he takes my hand. "Breathe into it." Gradually the pain and tears subside as he strokes my hand, looking with concern into my eyes. When I'm somewhat calmer he inserts the second needle into my other calf. It too is painful, but I am able to breathe into it and the moment is quickly past.

Now he proceeds to my chest, which feels like a clenched fist turned in on itself. With his deft fingers he gently explores the tensions there, massaging a little. Then the needle goes in. I let out a howl as my tense body doubles up in agony. My naked torso contracts violently around the sharp fire in my chest.

"Breathe into it," he says for the second time. I hear his calm voice from far away. I seem to be staring into a volcano at night, darkness and fire closing in around me. I am sobbing violently, clutching his arm. Gradually, I become aware of his other arm supporting my head and back. I try to relax a little, but breathing more deeply brings another wave of excruciating pain. I cry out uncontrollably, realizing that the dam that has held all this tension and grief for so long, is crumbling.

He's right there with me, compassionate, supporting. But he doesn't take the needle out. I am acutely aware of my naked chest. Feel too exposed. My sobs are like the howls of a wounded, wild animal. Uncontrollable, wrenching, ancient, raw. Irrational outrage mixed with relief. Blood splattered on the face of the moon. He continues to hold me while the sobs alternate with attempts to relax into the needle.

Finally, the fire begins to subside. My head drops back exhausted into the support of his arm. My clenched spine begins to uncurl against his gentle body. Slowly my back releases, returning me once more to the waiting table. He takes my hand as my arm comes to rest once more by my side. I feel his other hand stroking my forehead. Calm. Gentle.

A snowy egret suddenly fills my mind's eye, standing serene at water's edge. I feel her quietly watching me.

"I didn't want to alarm everybody," I whimper through my remaining tears, aware of how loud my sobbing and shrieks have been, how much louder they might have grown had I not felt constrained by the nearness of strangers.

"They'll understand," he murmurs reassuringly. "We all have emotions." His eyes search mine.

"You are so kind," I whisper as a new wave of tears takes hold of me.

A long pause passes between us while he holds my hand and watches my eyes with his own unobtrusive but fully present gaze.

Finally I grow quiet.

"Has it been awhile since you cried?"

"It's been weeks."

"I'm going to give you an herbal remedy that should help your lungs, and may also help with the depression. I'll leave you to rest now. I'll be back soon to take out the needles."

"O.K.," I respond weakly. The needles are no longer painful. They are silently doing their work. I let myself sink into the support of the table. My mind, mercifully, goes blank.

I rest, still feeling vulnerable and exposed, like a baby, like a lover, aware of the intimacy that has just passed between us.

This gentle, straight man passionately in love with his two-year-old son, his daughter, his wife, his work, his life. Seasoned meditator, committed healer, old, old soul. Man of herbs and needles profound with compassion.

And me, his contemporary, a gay man living with and most probably dying of AIDS, carrying the grief of a community under siege, lying nearly naked on a table in a darkened cubicle between walls too thin to contain my cries. No shirt to cover my aching heart. Bare feet and calves. Clothed only in jeans rolled up to my knees. I feel too exposed. I could not have handled being totally naked. Not now. Not yet.

Too much like death, like a stiff on a slab.

And curiously, too much like birth. I am both drawn and repelled by the image of complete helplessness. To be totally naked, totally dependent. Totally and completely at the mercy of others.

There is a part of me that wants desperately to surrender, to be stripped of ambition, to let go of this world and the cares of this body, to abandon all responsibility and striving. I feel like a little boy wanting to reach up and have the adult's sure, loving hand close around mine and lead me on. I am tired of being my own adult. I long to stop thinking. I would love to give up this obsession for meaning that insists upon wrestling some blessing out of every dark angel that bars the road. It is a child's dream, to be so carefree. Or an old man's, to be released. It is the desire to abdicate. To give up responsibility that can only be mine.

But it is also the soul's cry for home.

Mixed in with the seductive urge to give up, is a very real need to surrender. The impulse to reach up my little hand to seek comfort and guidance from a bigger hand is not merely a childish wish for escape. It is a deep, sacred impulse, an acknowledgment of the need to trust something bigger than the little "I". I long to lay down my mind and body on some ancient and yet quite contemporary altar, where fire can consume all that is inessential.

But where is that altar? How do I let go?

I need more time. I am not ready yet. I'm not prepared to lie naked, even among healers, to surrender that completely, to trust that much. I am not prepared to give up my body and mind. It is not yet time.

But I am nearly ready to surrender my soul. I need to let go.

But how?

In one powerful gesture of wings, the egret explodes into awesome flight. Its wavering image still cleaves to the water, growing smaller and smaller as the bird ascends.

Please, just give me a little more time. I'm getting ready as fast as I can. I still need my body. I still need my mind. I cannot or will not let go of my last shred of armor. I am not ready to be stripped bare.

Soon, but not now. Soon, but not yet.

Coming Home Hospice

DARK FOG ROLLS DOWN over the freeway as I make the approach to the city from the north. I shut the vents in the truck and turn on the heat. San Francisco has always refused to be predictable. The bridge is enshrouded as I reach it. Ill-clad tourists stroll stoically across, doing what they'd come to do, taking each other's pictures against a backdrop of rust-colored cables rising into the mist like severed arteries vainly pumping life into thin air.

Bill is slipping fast. He has been in the Hospice now for two weeks. Trying to talk with him by phone has proven to be an exercise in frustration. He sounds drugged and can't find most of the words he wants. His pauses between words have become so long I think he's forgotten I'm on the line. "Bill," I shout loudly into the wires. "Bill, are you there?"

"Hello?" he finally manages, tentative, confused and ill-defined like the prow of a little boat struggling to emerge through the fog.

"I'm coming to see you. I'll be there tomorrow."

Another long pause.

"Bill, are you listening? I'll see you tomorrow. I have to go now."

Silence on the other end. I can hear him breathing.

"Well good-bye then. I love you." I hang onto the receiver a little while longer.

Finally his wavering voice comes over the wire. "O.K.," he says wistfully, sounding uncertain as to what or with whom he may have agreed.

"I love you sweetheart. I'll see you tomorrow."

I hang up the receiver and stare out the window numb and shocked, knowing there will be no more phone calls. I didn't know he had lost so much ground.

▼ ▼ ▼ ▼ ▼

A discreet brass plaque attached to the large wooden door announces "Coming Home Hospice". An old converted convent in the heart of the Castro. The door is locked. I ring the bell and wait. In a minute or two a chubby woman with a quick smile appears and lets me in, and then as suddenly disappears, I suppose assuming that I've been here before and know my way around. We exchange no words. There is a visitors' log in a prominent location on a desk just inside the door. I do as the others have done, signing my name and the time of my arrival. Then I look around. I am in a little entrance area with a hall leading off and a staircase ascending to the second floor. It is very quiet, except for an occasional moan or inarticulate cry coming from above. I climb the stairs. Another hall. I walk past several rooms, all with open doors. One is filled with gregarious Latinos clustered around a friend. In other rooms patients are sleeping or staring out as I pass by. The moaning grows louder, closer. I glance quickly into the room where a moaning man is thrashing in pain, a nurse busy replacing an I.V. bag. I wince and pass by.

Finally, I find Bill. Again I am shocked. His skull is protruding through his sunken face. He appears to be asleep. He lies in bed straight as an arrow, perfectly centered. His long, thin fingers are folded together, resting on the single blanket covering his slender body. He has always been utterly organized, in control, nothing lax or out of place. I wonder if he's really asleep, or is just resting with his eyes closed.

"Bill," I whisper.

His large dark eyes open and look over at me. "Hi, honey," he says without smiling.

"How are you?" No response. His face is a blank. "Are you dying?"

"Hmph!" he exclaims, shutting his eyes and turning his head away, back to his perfectly centered position.

Stupid, stupid question! Of course he's dying! How could I make such a blunder? I don't know how to do this. I sit empty and shut out next to his bed, wishing I had simply said, "I love you." Or been silent.

Time passes. His eyes open. He stares straight ahead at the blank wall as though he is watching something there. I have the strong sense that whatever he looks at is on the other side; his eyes aren't seeing anything here right now. His brow furrows and he seems disturbed, confused when footsteps pass in the hall or the front doorbell rings.

After a while, he raises a hand as if to scratch an itch on the side of his face. His hand stays suspended in the air next to his face, not scratching. It just stays there. It seems so strange, and I have trouble letting it be.

Finally I say, "Would you like some help getting your hand down?" He looks over at me and then at his hand.

"How did it get there?" he asks.

"You had an itch," I tell him.

"Oh," he says and lowers the hand back down to fold in with the other again. His eyes close as he returns to his perfectly centered position.

I wait awhile longer and sense that this time he's really sleeping. I've been here about an hour. I'm ready to leave. I bend over and kiss his bony forehead. He doesn't stir. "Good-bye, Bill," I whisper. "I love you."

This was harder than I expected. I'm glad to get away. I am relieved as the big oak door closes behind me and I am blasted by the chilled, foggy air so comfortingly familiar from all the years I lived in the city. I stand for a long moment indecisively on the sidewalk, until I start to chill. I'm not ready to go home, not ready to turn my back on the city and head for sunny Sonoma County. I want the cold air and this gay neighborhood where similar dramas to Bill's are being played out all around me. I am part of this sub-culture. I have lived and worked here. I know these men. My feet instinctively carry me down the few blocks to 18th and Castro, turn up Castro and stumble into Welcome Home where I've eaten many a country dinner, especially when I was single. It really is a bit like coming home. Pleasant country decor. Nice waiters. Good food.

I find a corner table. "Just a cup of coffee."

"Sure," says the veteran waiter. He's been here for years. I can tell from his kind voice that he knows what I'm going through. He's seen it all before, too many times.

He returns with the coffee, pours me a cup. "Now you take your time, honey."

Sometimes a kind waiter is better than therapy. I start to breathe a little as the warmth of this old, familiar restaurant and this simple cup of coffee begin to cradle me and distance me from the shock of seeing Bill in such decline.

As I start to thaw a little, I realize how lonely it is here. Not yet dinner time, the few other patrons sit singly at tables, like me. No couples. No conversations. A little too quiet.

Coming Home. Welcome Home. Strangers in little rooms moaning or staring. Strangers at little tables drinking coffee, like me. Nurses and waiters tending to the fragile. These tables used to be more comforting when I had nowhere else to go. Now there's Conrad and Petaluma and real earth and trees. Life in abundance. Life waiting for me. Even though I'm filled with sadness, I am ready to go home. A different kind of home from hospices and restaurants. An earthly home. A warm house and lover, a cat and a garden, a place with a past, a present and a future. It is there that my welcome awaits.

I am on my way home.

Oh, dear Bill, you are already on your way out. We barely connected there at the Hospice, unlike all the previous times. Before, you were always happy to see me, and this time I felt irrelevant, even a little resented, calling you back into a reality you are in the process of leaving. I felt inadequate, so inept. Why couldn't I have just sat quietly and channeled love and light to you? Why couldn't I have put aside my own need to be recognized and loved by you? I have grown used to your face lighting up when I entered your room, so it was a shock to receive no smile, no reaching out of your hand. Perhaps I should have reached for yours. Yet you seemed so self-contained, so much like a monk in deep contemplation, that I'm sure it would have been an unwelcome intrusion. It was too hard to leave you this way, too sad.

I leave the restaurant, thanking the kind waiter on my way out, walk up the cold and windy street to the truck, climb gratefully into it, and head for home.

Gentle Rain

"Fall is such a beautiful space
To shed the old with love and grace."

— MARTHA IMBERG

THE FIRST GENTLE RAIN of the season is falling softly
against the windows. Individual droplets gather on the
glass, pausing in their travels as though to look in on the
warm lamplight gentling me here in the grey morning,
before they merge and slide down the glass in sad, slow
rivulets. I have been told that in native traditions the
recently departed come back as rain; that the gentlest
showers are "female rain" and that the hard, driving rain
is "male." However that may be, against our windows this
morning the gentlest of rains is falling.

Martha is gone. She died yesterday. Bob called in the
afternoon to give me the news. She died close to noon, at
home like she wanted to, baby-sitting her one-and-a-half
year-old granddaughter Christa. "My angel," she called
her.

It appears that Martha had been trying to make lunch
in the kitchen and had struggled to the bedroom where
she collapsed on her bed, perhaps trying to dial 911, perhaps deciding not to make the call. Christa's father John
discovered them at three o'clock when he came to take
Christa home. The front door was locked and there was no
response to the doorbell. He could hear Christa crying in
the house, so he pried off the screen and came through

the window into Martha's room, where he found her lying on her bed.

Bob was at work in Santa Rosa. Friends came to be with him through the late afternoon after he came home. I sat with him in the evening while he made his phone calls. "She's free at last!" he exclaimed, his arms shooting up into the air. "She went straight for the light like an arrow, I know it. This was her last incarnation. She was ready to go!"

I, too, feel the relief of her release from her body. She had survived the doctors' predictions of demise for nearly ten years. She lived with a heart so badly damaged by cardiomyopathy that professionals just shook their heads at the X-rays and told her, "You shouldn't be alive. We don't understand it." Diabetes and sleep apnea added to her difficulties in the final months. She was on eighteen different medications. They filled up half a large shopping bag when Bob collected them and threw them all away.

"I have two hearts," Martha once explained. "It's as though my physical heart is made of tin, all rusty and failing, while my true heart just keeps growing stronger and stronger." All of us who knew her felt the truth of that statement. Martha was the biggest-hearted person I have ever had the privilege to know. To love and be loved by her was one of the great gifts of my life.

She was easily and often moved to tears. Her emotions were like the shifting patches of light and shade playing among the leaves of a widespread maple tree blazing gold in autumn. Her eyes would grow large and she'd say, "Oh my God!" when someone else might have said "uh-huh" in response. She made me feel like my stories really mattered, that I really mattered. We met every week during the last months of her life. How we both treasured our brief time together! After her hospitalization in July, I drove her each week to our Monday night meeting, and we shared our stories and feelings as the landscape rambled past.

Martha is gone. She left yesterday. Last night the wind was so strong, it rattled the windows and made the shades in our bedroom slap and sigh against the frames. "Are you out there?" I whispered, sitting up in bed. It was useless trying to sleep, I felt so charged with her energy. I crept out of bed silently so as not to disturb Conrad, ran a hot bath and lit the room full with candles. In the bathtub, for hours I read *The Tibetan Book of Living and Dying* that Martha had lent me, and found myself singing chants for her I had never heard before: "Om Shri Rama." Over and over I intoned on a resonant low note, a slow, consistent, joyous outpouring of sound. (Bob told me later that Om is the universal sacred sound, that Shri means "praise," and that Rama is a powerful manifestation of the godhead as the Archer.)

Rama had particular significance for Martha. It was through archery that she first experienced herself as powerful, capable, worthy. Like so many other women and men in this culture, she had been abused as a child. It was during her first marriage that she started to discover her real abilities through archery. She had taken up the bow and arrow at the prompting of her husband, who subsequently resented her when her abilities surpassed his. She studied hypnosis to perfect her powers of concentration, later offering classes in her home to help other women, becoming so successful in archery competitions that the judges felt it was no longer fair for her to compete with women. So she entered the men's competition and won! She told me how she shot a bull's-eye dead center in the target. Her second arrow lodged in the shaft of the first. Her third and final arrow split the second asunder. Martha was a straight shooter. Once she set her will, there was little that could stop her.

She asked her doctor once if it was wise for her to travel. "Absolutely not!" he declared. The next day she left on a pilgrimage to India. "I may have been sick in bed the whole time," she later confided, "but at least I was sick in *India!* "

She worked with disabled children and young adults, by all reports doing her job brilliantly without benefit of formal training. She loved those kids in a way few of us are ever loved; profoundly, deeply, and with an intuitive sense of what each child really needed. She made astonishing progress with the "problem children" others had given up on. "Those kids became my most loyal friends after I became too sick to continue working," she told me. "They called. They visited. They sent me love letters."

A week before Martha made her transition, she said that she knew she would soon be leaving.

"How long do you think you have?" I asked her.

"Two to six months. Maybe less."

"If you do die soon, is there anything you need from me before you go?" I felt profoundly serene as I asked her that question, a serenity that came from somewhere far beyond my own need and emotions. Our hands rested softly in each other's.

"I want you to do my memorial service," she said through her tears. "I've been waiting for the right person to come along. I think that's why you were sent to me."

I felt humbled and honored, and told her so. We sat for a long time just gazing at each other, holding onto each other's hands.

"Do you have any unfinished business?" I asked her the next day.

"No," she said, looking up through moist eyes as we sat

close together on her big blue sofa. As usual, her pugs snuggled up against us, Angel and Baby lying at her feet, Rocky just above us on the back of the sofa with his tongue hanging out and his bright eyes bulging. How she loved those dogs! And children. And life. "No, I have no unfinished business. I feel very complete with everyone, very current."

Martha had called the funeral home just the day before to make arrangements for her cremation. "That's too expensive!," she insisted to the undertaker, until he admitted the availability of a long cardboard box. "That'll be fine," she'd told him. "I don't need anything fancy."

Martha was complete. There were no loose ends.

She was concerned most for Bob, knowing what a huge loss her leaving would be for him. She was relieved that Conrad and I had come into their lives and felt that we would be a big help to Bob. "It's hardest to leave the children, especially little Christa," she said, squeezing my hand hard. "She's such an unusual child. She's been like a guide and companion to me." Christa was Martha's first grandchild, Lisa's daughter, fruit of her fruit. Her second grandchild was born the week that she died. Life continuing. New life emerging.

Martha's brother Lother died less than a month ago. She was determined to make it to his memorial service in Grass Valley, fully realizing that she could die making the effort. Once more the doctors warned against travel, particularly to such a high altitude. Martha arranged for Lother's son and his girlfriend, a hospice nurse, to come for her, driving her up Monday and back Tuesday night in a van in which she could lie down.

I talked to her Wednesday morning after she returned home. She was radiant with enthusiasm over the phone. The trip had gone extremely well, and there were no physical crises to interfere with the flow of love Martha and her family felt for each other. "I didn't realize I had affected so many people," she confided in me. One distant relative told her she had been so moved by Martha's stories of the special children Martha had worked with that she, herself, became a foster parent to four children. The celebration of Lother's life afforded a celebration of Martha's life as well while she was still alive. She learned on that trip just how many lives had been touched by her loving heart. She came home as radiant, complete and whole as any of us could hope to be before we die.

That was two days ago. Now she's gone. How do I feel? Numb. Scared of the responsibility I've taken on, to lend comfort and support to Bob and the other family and friends I have not yet met. Will I be loving enough? Present enough? You deserve the best, Martha. I will do the best I can.

I'll miss you, Martha. I'll miss your passion, your love, your profound understanding. I have had few friends who seemed to "get" who I am as thoroughly and compassionately as you did, even at our first meeting. I'll miss as well giving what I was able to give you, and your gratitude at receiving it. I'll miss your deep need and ability to trust so well, even after an early life that proved brutally untrustworthy. I'll miss being your neighbor, calling you when I'm confused or happy and hearing your pleasure at my call rush over the wires to embrace me. I'll miss dropping in for iced tea, the long hours on your couch, the wildly enthusiastic greeting I always received from Rocky and Baby, leaping and licking before settling down with old Angel, too blind and deaf to know who I was. I'll miss our drives through the country and your hand holding mine.

I will miss you, Martha.

But precious, beloved friend, I'm glad that you are free.

With Bob, I share the image of you shooting straight into the Light, perfectly concentrated on the center of your goal. I know that you're gone, but I feel your energy continuing strongly. Continuing to bless us and love us and encourage us to live on with honesty, passion and courage.

How do I feel? I feel profoundly blessed. I feel sad and joyful all jumbled up together. I feel like running and weeping, like dancing in circles. I feel like phoning you, Martha, to share my elation and my sadness. I turn to dial, and then remember that you're gone. For a moment I don't know what to do. How can you be gone when you feel so present? Is it possible I will never hear your voice again?

Your friendship is a treasure I will never forget. How do I feel? I feel like one of the luckiest people on earth to have had a friend such as you. Go well, my dear, into that bright night. You are, indeed, a child of the Light.

Rain down, gentle rain, rain down.

Baptism

OH BILLY, YOU'RE GONE NOW TOO, just three days after Martha and Doug. When will it stop?

I'm sitting here holding your picture, the one from our trip to the river where you are smiling so broadly as you look up from collecting brown weeds in sunshine. I'm sitting here holding you—missing you—wanting you. Never again to see that smile, to hear you laugh or speak or play the piano. Never again to feel your lithe body hugging me with such tenderness and quiet strength. Never again to watch the ocean together, or the clouds, or to sit over coffee at city cafes watching the people.

I remember the first and last time I whispered into your ear, "I love you. I want you in my life." You held me back at arm's length and with that ironic and tolerant expression you had, you said simply, "Well, here I am!" Then you laughed and shoved me away gently and I felt kindly chided for being too sentimental. Strange how with a word or a look you could make me feel silly and a bit exposed, but at the same time loved and appreciated for the very foibles you never allowed yourself. You allowed yourself very few indulgences. I think you could have been happy as a monk. So self-contained. So discreet with words. So well practiced in meditation and acceptance.

I hold your dear image here in my hand and the memory of that happier day at the river comes flooding back to me. You stand proudly clutching those brown weeds in your sensitive city hands. You are wearing a white polo shirt and green-rimmed dark glasses. Behind you is that incredible blue, blue sky. I remember a warm sun pouring out of that sky. A glorious, perfect Fall day.

Six years ago now, almost to the day. Do you remember, dear Bill, that first trip to the country together, our retreat at The Willows on the river? Autumn, my favorite time of year. Morning, my favorite time of day. My mind wanders back to the delicious pleasures of that morning at The Willows.

The river was still in shadow from the tall redwood trees rising into bright sky across from our bedroom perch. Split-pea green where the sun dappled the dark velvet, almost black in the shadows along the opposite bank. Sun warm through the open windows, aqua-green and lace curtains tucked aside to reveal the view and let in the morning. Windows wide to the morning sounds of piano in the parlor, country traffic from the old river road, remote barking, bird-song and occasional lazy voices floating up from the deck below, all mingled and dreamy, coming in like the sound of an easy surf at the windows of an ocean cottage.

I was propped on pillows with the mugged decaf and muffins you had brought me from below, still in an altered state of grace from our recent love-making. The memory is fresh and sweet, of light spilling all around and seemingly through us, embracing a miracle of souls embodied and at one. You, so slender, still with a dancer's body at age forty-two. Me, like a gentle mountain of rising and falling passions covered with bracken and moss, more bear than man, wild and woodsy, just turning forty.

You had gone below again to read the paper in the sun and slough off another layer of loosening city skin. I lay moored there on our island·bed musing through green curtains of taffeta, then willow, following my eyes' mystic journey down the long, open lawn, past the preening ducks to the dark watery finger of velvet beyond, dark green flecked with floating yellow leaves and dashes of sunlight.

Finally I arose from reverie and assembled myself, happy in the knowledge that there was nothing we needed to do, no place we needed to be. After more coffee and muffins on the deck, we decided to take out the canoe to adventure upstream.

I remember watching you as you happily gathered brown weeds on the little knoll where we landed the canoe, beaching it loosely without tying up on the grassy bank a mile or so upriver from The Willows. I followed you closely through my camera lens, intent on getting at least one good picture of you out of my roll of thirty-six. You allowed me my obsession without paying me much mind, like a yawning lion tolerates the attentions of a safari of tourists.

The warm sun kept trying to get my attention. Several times I almost put the camera down, almost let the sun's perfect warmth take me over. Almost sank down into the grassy embrace of the slope and let myself melt into the dazzling light all around us. Almost drifted up into the blue sky above. Almost. But I couldn't quite let go of my compulsive mission. Our intimacy was still fledgling, not quite secure. A part of me wanted to catch you and preserve you somehow the same way I tried to capture the elusive beauty of butterflies as a child by netting them and pinning them down.

So I tracked you carefully with my camera, at a bit of a distance, recording everything I saw: the river behind you, your hands full of weeds, your enigmatic smile in a face with eyes hidden behind those dark glasses. And I insisted that you take a picture of me, eyes closed in the grass, pretending to be at one with it all. Even in the picture I look like a fraud.

I think in fact I *did* finally see you gathering your weeds. Still walking like the city boy you've always been, stepping high to be sure of clearance in the grass, you nevertheless seemed to merge with your gathering, your smile softening in concentrated meditation, your fine wrinkles wrinkling around the edges of the green frames, your fastidious hands carefully breaking the stems and holding your collection. All over and around the green knoll you clambered like a beaver cutting saplings to weave into security of home before Winter.

We climbed back into the canoe and continued our adventure upstream. And then, do you remember, all the weeds were gone. The pictures gone. Your glasses gone. My favorite suede moccasins gone. All gone into the river where the rapids played with us and dumped us out. "We're going to hit!" I yelled to you and the next thing I knew I was being swept along by the river, trying to reach the surface without losing the boat or the oars, hoping that you knew how to swim, not seeing you anywhere as I came to the surface. Finally you emerged sputtering on the other side of the boat.

It had seemed so shallow and tame from the canoe. We kept scraping bottom in a gentle kind of way. Just a lazy Autumn idyll. But not here! Here it was wild and wet and rapid. My bare feet painfully struck bottom as the river swept us under and up and along.

All of our tokens of the river were dumped out and drowned, all the ways we had tried to capture the experience without getting wet. All the lenses we had looked through to frame and focus and filter were swamped or swept away. Plunged to the murky bottom with bare feet and alarm, we were everywhere embraced by green rushing fingers playing with our bodies like a skilled and laughing lover, tugging at our clothes, the oars, the canoe, stripping us of anything loose enough to sink or float away.

And so it happened, unexpected, profound—this shaking off of shackles that had held me prisoner within myself, unable to merge, to feel my true connection with all that was around me, unable to dissolve into the greater Being.

We had dutifully watched the river's reflections, exclaimed at the golden maples, slept in the luscious big bed, eaten the excellent muffins, greeted the intelligent guests, leafed through the lovely books, examined the outlandishly costumed fish in the anemone tank, lounged before the crackling fire, submerged in the sensuous hot tub and emerged and gazed at a black sky full of stars.

But none of it had touched the emptiness I had been carrying during the recent months of loss. It couldn't bring Kenneth back, or Joan, or Wayne. Touch down in this river of loss at any point—the names change, but the grief itself becomes like a river, ongoing, each new grief a swell merging with the griefs that have gone before. We're lucky to get a break of a few months between losses. Some of us have lost everyone we cared for. None of this country-inn luxury had quieted my fears for my parents' increasing vulnerability at the hands of old age, doctors and disease. Nor could it reverse the fact of the virus quietly going about its business in these bodies I love, yours and mine, and in dozens more I cherish whose owners have broken bread with me. None of it answered the deep unnamed questions I hardly knew how to ask.

What is happening to us? Is there meaning in all this disease and dying?

In loving, we open ourselves to loss.

But oh, not to love is too sad, too lonely to bear. Life, death, community, quality of life—these are our issues, but the real question lies buried below the level of words, stored in our very sinews like a howl or a wordless prayer. We ache for an answer to a question so deep and universal we cannot begin to name it.

But the river understood the question and knew the answer and like the sudden slap of a Zen master's rod, it dumped us out and hugged us under just long enough for us to experience the answer. It only took a moment to shake us loose, remove our bonds and leave us finally free again.

As soon as we'd bobbed to the surface, located each other through the blur of green, rescued the oars and seen that my shoes and your glasses and lovely weeds were gone and my camera and checkbook and your wallet were all pocketed under water, then we looked at each other and just started to laugh. And we went on laughing uncontrollably. After we'd figured out how to right the canoe and get ourselves back into it we floated back down river like two bedraggled rats. And whenever one or the other of us would burst again into laughter, we both just filled up with it and our laughter *was* the sun, *was* the river, *was* the reason we had come.

We tie up the canoe at the Willows dock, cross the long lawn and sneak into our room undetected. The late afternoon sun is slanting in the window as we dress for dinner.

It is all green here. The willows, the redwoods, the curtains, the shirt I'm wearing to dinner tonight, the lawn, the leaves on the river, the river itself. All green and shades of green, with honeyed light everywhere. Across the lawn, through the window, embracing the clean sheets, illuminating your red-brown moustache and pale skin, pinks and browns and russets and golds all swimming together before me like leaves swirling in a sun-lit eddy. Light warms your dark lustrous hair where my grateful hand grazes its little flock of fingers as you pull on your socks. Light plays in your sweet smile wrinkling up with pleasure and in your hazel eyes as you turn your long, lovely body toward me to embrace. There is light everywhere. In our room. In the river. In us. So much light! And green—every shade of beautiful green!

There is almost no tomorrow. Almost no last day before we have to head home. There is almost, only, the memory of green and a river full of sunlight and laughter.

But life continues and death is part of life's dance.

Go well, dear friend to wherever you are flowing. May the Great River guide you and see you on. You gave me much. Your quietude. Your subtle humour. Your care as to a younger brother. I miss your wisdom and spiritual strength. I miss you, dear man. How not?

It is nearly more than I can bear, this string of deaths of dear friends in such a short time. It will be some time before I register all the feelings that have been shaking my world the last few days. For now, I am glad for some comfort. Grace has permitted me this picture of you, salvaged from the long, wet roll. As I sit here holding what's left of you, the sun finds your image and lights up your face. I can almost see your deep brown eyes laughing as you look out at me through those dark, green-rimmed glasses. They're gone in the river.

And now you, too, are gone.

Gently Now

Gently now
The small things done well
The cat fed
The garden tended

Grief

I HAVE BEEN STRUGGLING to keep despair at bay. I have not been able to write in weeks. I am both afraid to and drawn to give in to the depression that has been hounding me this past month or so. Afraid that depression will lead to despair. From despair the step over the line back into addiction would be so easy and so utterly devastating, destroying everything I have worked so hard to claim over the past thirteen years of recovery. Self-esteem, the ability to trust, to love, to show up and tell the truth, overcoming fear in order to make a living, finally supporting myself and even contributing money to helping others, rediscovering a belief in some benevolent energy beyond myself, the incomparable, precious gift of community, the ability to forgive and be forgiven. All, all so easily lost if despair takes hold and shame shuts the people who would love me out of my life. I do not want to revert to that place of desperate misery ever again.

Yet the mental energy it takes to return again and again to a hopeful, positive perspective is exhausting. Many times recently I have wanted to just give up, give in to the depression and even to despair. I want to and perhaps need to let go into darkness. Like Persephone sinking into an annual Hades, I must make the journey down again before I can embody an authentic Spring.

I have been flailing to keep my head above water while below the surface my body and the bodies of my friends are being eaten alive by sharks. Three deaths last week,

Doug, Martha and Bill. Charlie's partner Tom diagnosed again with Pneumocystis, Jessica dying of cancer in Santa Fe. Six more members of our Gay Men's Spiritual Retreat community are gone since our last gathering as many months ago. It is hard to catch your breath before another is gone. I need to grieve. The tears are frozen behind my ribs.

I do not cry alone. I need a life-line back to the surface if I am to surrender to the teeth of the sharks. I am interviewing therapists, grief counselors, body workers. I need help. One support group a week is not enough right now, and the talk there is all about choosing the light. There's not much room for the darkness.

With a life-line in place, with someone who is not afraid of the dark, I believe I could and would go down. The sharks will not destroy me utterly. They may even prove to be servants of the truth, teeth of the gods, tearing away the non-essentials, ripping open my grief-filled heart. There are so many tears pounding against my ribs. My chest aches, longing to release them. I want to sink down. I want to let go.

Friends offer hope, new therapies, new books. *You Don't Have to Die, Surviving With AIDS*. I have been able to incorporate some of the information, make changes in my diet, pursue meditation, continue with support groups. But there is too much advice, too many new books, too many hopeful therapies and promising news articles.

Conrad was sitting cross-legged on the window-bench reading the Sunday paper yesterday morning when I got up. He was excited by an article about blood transfusions from healthy HIV-positive patients to those not doing so well. Test results seemed promising. He read several sections out loud to me while I stood obedient and numb, gazing out the window unseeingly past him into the garden. I could not muster a positive response. I was relieved to get away to another room, out of range of the news, away from hope and advice.

I do not want hope. Not right now. I am tired of trying to juggle a commitment to life with preparation for death. I feel like a marionette being jerked back on stage just when I was adjusting to being dumped in the wings. I resent the strings that pull me back. Expectations from friends that I will "fight the good fight," responsibilities to a home and a lover, a cat, a garden. I find myself resenting the latest enthusiasm of the well-meaning who presume, I suppose, that I want to recover. I don't. I want a little longer. That's all. I want to write these words and tell my story through the coming Winter and Spring, a year of seasons—it is enough. I only need my health a little longer. I need to make my will and clear out my files and shelves, give away a few things to those who might enjoy them. And then, perhaps then, I can finally stop.

There is not that much holding me here. My commitment to Conrad, yes. He has already been abandoned once by losing a lover to AIDS. I wish I could spare him. But what really does it matter if I live an extra year or two? Whenever I go, he will miss me and be forced once more to grieve his losses, to decide himself whether to check-out or continue. What does it matter if I leave next Spring or five or more Summers or Winters from now?

The strings are loosening, being cut. Three more last week. Doug, Martha, Bill. I was committed to Bill and also to Martha. I had already let go of Doug, knowing he was surrounded by closer friends, feeling the truth of my own limitations, allowing a phone call to suffice where before I would have proposed a visit. But for Martha and Bill, I was still showing up, holding hands, listening to their wisdom and fears, reminding them of the loving beings they are, sharing with them both the glory and the pain of transition. They were important teachers to me. Both had struggled and learned for over ten years at the feet of their respective gurus and life-threatening conditions. They were both exceptional, long-term survivors. Now they're gone. There is a large part of me that wants to go with them, into the unknown, away from here.

I'm scared at the thought that I might survive. It is the same fear I had several years ago when I realized that I would rather die than become a lonely, impoverished and marginalized old man. I accepted the challenge of that realization, raised my landscaping rates, and made a commitment to my old man by opening my first I.R.A. account. I made a commitment to live. I believed I could survive. I had done well for so long. I got busy to ensure a reasonably comfortable future. I believed that if I had money and had not lost my soul, I would have friends, even as an old man. Family and friends aligned themselves with my stated belief that I would be a survivor.

The bout with Pneumocystis last summer and my subsequent decision to go on disability have changed things considerably. I dissolved my I.R.A. accounts as part of the "spending down" necessary to qualify for benefits. I "sheltered" money in a friend's account. At the advice of friends, I stopped working myself and continued only with the bare necessities of scheduling and billing to keep a maintenance crew in the field taking care of the gardens we've built. I dismantled the structure that had been a symbol of my faith and my hope that I might still be here when this epidemic is over. Now where is my belief in the possibility of longevity? Where is my commitment to continuing on? What will become of the old man if I do survive, now that the I.R.A.'s are gone? Have I stopped the exhausting juggling act that has kept the two possible scenarios for my life up in the air? Survival to old age or death at the hands of AIDS? Have I really made a decision to move towards death? In so many ways it is the easier choice.

Who will be left if I do survive? Everyone's leaving. I long to go too. Who will help me descend into Hades? Is my rage buried there among the ashes of friends? Where are my feelings? Where is my grief?

The sharks are striking, pulling me down. Finally down into a sea of tears.

Letter to Gay Men's Spiritual Retreat Community

Dear Friends and Sacred Brothers,

Bill Alvis died peacefully at Coming Home Hospice on Sunday, September 25. His long-time living companion, Bhavo Michaels, and several other close friends and family members were with him through the process of his accelerated decline in health over the past year. Severe neuropathy, sinus problems, dehydration and weight loss left him hospitalized on several occasions in recent months. In July, Bill was diagnosed with dementia. Despite the diagnosis, he remained lucid for the most part, and recognized family and friends right up until the end. But communication became more and more of a struggle as he searched, sometimes in vain, for elusive words. We spent an afternoon in August while he was still living at home labeling drawers and shelves in his room so he could more easily remember what everything was called. Shortly after that time together, Bill was admitted to the Psych. ward at St. Mary's Hospital, where he stayed several weeks before being transferred to the AIDS Ward, and then in his final weeks to Coming Home Hospice. Toward the end it became increasingly more difficult for him to complete sentences, respond to questions, or focus his attention on the outer world.

Having been treated successfully for lymphadenopathy in 1981, Bill was a long-term survivor with AIDS who was an inspiration and source of hope and wisdom to those of us who knew him well. Bill was an accomplished pianist and had worked both as an accompanist and music critic in his younger days in New York. In more recent years he worked in the Surveillance Department of the AIDS wing of the San Francisco Department of Public Health, where his caring, funny, knowledgeable presence was a cherished cohesive energy for the staff.

Bill and I met while singing together in The Pacific Chamber Singers which performed AIDS benefit concerts for several years in the late eighties and early nineties. It was during this period that I introduced Bill to GMSR.

Bill was a generally reserved and, at times, intensely private person, deeply engaged by classical music and enjoying long hours at the piano alone. He was also committed and deeply informed by a long-standing meditation practice that had guided him for many years. He dressed most frequently in black or dark green. They were colors that suited him.

We'll miss you, Bill. In a world chaotic with distractions and diversions, thank you for your lessons of self-containment, acceptance and quiet passion.

With love and cherished memories, both of Bill and of you, my other sacred brothers both living and passed on. May we continue to be reservoirs of love and light for each other. May we continue to provide each other with safe harbor, where we can discover and express our deepest feelings and most complete truths. May we continue to honor each other in our splendid diversity. From profound silliness to profound sorrow, may we continue to risk exposing all the facets of this incredible rainbow of light that enfolds us and renews us every time we gather in mourning, in visioning, in play.

With much love
"until we meet again."
Duncan

Collapsing Sunflowers

THE SUNFLOWERS ARE COLLAPSING under the weight of their own seed. Their tattered leaves hang withered, brittle brown rags that rattle in the least bit of wind. For weeks they have been leaning out further and further at ever more rakish angles towards the front of the border, away from the encroaching shade of the trees, seeking the sun. Only thirteen are still left standing and of these nearly half are bowed almost completely to the ground. The gardener in me wanted to stake them up to prevent their early demise, but I resisted the urge to interfere. The writer in me had made a commitment to observation without intervention.

But it proved too painful to let them lie broken and ruined after their fall. Of the original thirty-four, two thirds have crashed to the ground with broken stems. I have cut the stems back close to the ground, made a collection along the side of the garage of the seed-swollen heads, and returned leaves and stalks to the earth by way of the compost pile. It has been a season of sadness watching them come down.

The last of the sunflowers stand like ancient crones and withered old men, silently withessing the decline of their friends. Who would now believe that so recently they vibrated with the raw energy and green stuff of Summer, outstretched and alive, embracing the earth, the sky, the sun? They have lived well, fulfilled their destiny. They have completed what they came here to do.

My old friend, the strongest and tallest of the sunflowers, is still hanging on, bent over like a quiet old man, his head heavy with seed as though weighed down with too many memories. His last task in life is nearly complete, to bring the seed safely back down to earth.

A season of sadness watching them come down: Dewey Stewart, Michael del Villar, Martha Imberg, Bill Alvis, Doug DeBeni. They have already fallen. Others are bent over nearly to the ground, energy gradually ebbing away. Tom Mapp, George Kronenberger, Julio Suarez, Michael Tarpinian, Jessica Allen, Liz Cunningham, Don Struthers. Some may recover. Some no longer have the strength to bounce back. Their Summer is spent. Illness is claiming so many gentle souls. Who will be next? Who will be left?

Will the strongest and tallest last the season or crash down with the Fall? Who will still be here when the long Winter is over?

▼ ▼ ▼ ▼ ▼

It is Spring now. Only Julio and Michael have survived the Winter.

Fear of Winter

THE BRILLIANT LEAVES of the season are everywhere in evidence. Fiery liquidambers and Chinese pistachios are like bonfires blazing in the landscape. I love the yellow exclamation points of roadside poplars against the darker greens of redwoods and oaks. The way they break through the horizon of the earth to embrace the sky inspires me back into life, back from the edge of despair where I have recently stumbled so precariously.

Oh, there is still fear as the shadows lengthen. An ancient fear whispers in my blood as frost creeps out across the land. It is the fear of being caught out in the cold without protection, vulnerable to attacks by hungry wild things that rove the land in their various guises, stalking their prey singly or in desperate packs. It is the fear of being neither smart enough nor strong enough to stave off physical or spiritual assault by the forces of destruction. I fear being out of control. Being a victim. Being helpless. I fear being caught out too far from home.

"It is only fear," I remind myself. More often now I remember to breathe when the fear assails me. "It is only an old, historic fear. You don't have to give in to it."

But the despair that could yet claim me comes from an overwhelming season of sadness. A season of loss and grief. My sadness bears witness to much more than my own vulnerability, my illness, my dialogue with Death. What a precarious thing is life! My mind turns to the plight of those who have no home, those who are hungry.

The challenge of their lives intensifies as the days and nights grow colder and darker. The recent national and regional elections do not bode well for those in need. It seems we are entering yet darker times.

"Am I doing enough?" again I wonder. "Is it fair for me to experience happiness and contentment as long as there are endangered species, including my own, in our world, in my neighborhood?"

War, disease, loneliness, poverty. They sit huddled against my front door.

One of them has gotten in. He eats at our table and sleeps in our bed. His hollow eyes stare back at me in every room of the house. When I move, he moves. He probes the dark corridors and halls of my body. He is not content to be confined in one cramped cell. He ranges freely here and there. He knocks at locked doors inside my mind and gently but firmly demands entry. Like the snowy egret at the side of the road, he watches me dispassionately, observing my movements, body, mind and soul.

He poses a question. A hard question about life and connection. "What are you doing with this precious time?" "Are you loving well?" "Are you living fully?" "Will you be ready when it's time to let go?" It is the same question in different forms.

It is the question the seasons ask us again and again, making us aware of our deep-seated fears as the cold of Winter creeps in toward the hearth. Then at the very darkest hour, the seasons turn, awakening once more our hope, our faith, renewing once more our sense of openness and wonder as Spring slowly, inexorably renews the land. We try to protect ourselves from the changes by locking ourselves inside our houses and cars. We light up our supermarkets and offices so brightly, no shadow can lurk in an unexpected corner. Yet all the while Death is watching, courting our attention in a hundred different ways.

"Wake up!" Death whispers, as the leaves slide down, brushing against me, falling among the fading zinnias and carpeting the grass. "Wake up!" He whispers as I walk along the river and encounter the abandoned litter of the homeless, old mattresses and blankets, shopping carts, cardboard boxes and crates, here a doll, there a tiny shoe. Where have they gone, the men and women who assembled these livingrooms under the broad trees of Summer that now stand leafless in vacant lots, their tortured forms offering no protection against rain and raging winds?

My mind races back to the house. Have we done enough to prepare for Winter? I think of the woodpile neatly stacked within easy reach of the back door and the walnuts drying in the sun. I think of the well-built walls and insulated roof. I think of Conrad and our love for each other. I think of mornings with hot biscuits steaming from the oven and perhaps a friend or two stopped by to share them with us. I am reassured. We will last another Winter. But what about the others?

Life and Death are holding hands. They work long hours together, offering their lessons, posing their questions in a myriad of forms. Light and shadow in ever-shifting patterns play across the changing face of the land, trying to catch our attention, urging us to slow down and consider. "What are you doing with this precious time? Are you loving well? Are you living fully? Will you be ready when it's time to let go?"

The yellow poplars stand like prophets and evangelists in the landscape. "Prepare!" they warn. "Prepare!"

An Audience in Autumn

MY MIND IS SWIMMING with images of yellow leaves spiraling down through the blustery air into the river. The leafboats are finding their way to the sea. Conrad and I are spending an overnight in Rio Nido at The Village Inn, celebrating our third anniversary of meeting at Waller Bridge on a brilliant Fall day like today.

There is a tall maple tree here in Armstrong Woods that arches out over the outdoor amphitheater, against a backdrop of dark green redwoods. It reminds me of Martha. Blazing with passionate life. This was her favorite spot. She used to come here whenever she could, to be quiet. Bob buried her ashes behind the huge old General Sherman redwood where she spent hours meditating over the years. It's the perfect spot for her.

Conrad is up on the stage of the amphitheater and I am his only audience member in the very back row. I applaud wildly and call over to him, "Are you going to dance?" He does a bit of a jig and then pretends to fall into the orchestra pit. I gasp audibly with appropriate horror and cry out loudly, "Oh no!" After a time his head peeks over the edge of the pit. I feign great relief. Gradually his impish face emerges and then in one great leap he pops up over the edge to the audience level and stretches out his arms, presenting me with an eloquent bow. A lovely performance! More wild applause. He ambles back to where I am sitting and cozies in next to me. This man makes me happy. So very happy.

Winter is in the air. We both feel it. Time to seek out the comfort and pleasure awaiting us in the inn before going down to dinner.

Pumpkin Jam

LAST NIGHT CONRAD CUT UP THE JACK-O-LANTERNS and cooked up the pulp in a big stainless-steel pot on the stove. This morning he combined the pumpkin with raisins and apricots and lemons in a big, orange, cast-iron pot and left it simmering in the oven to cook down into jam.

"Could you stir it about every half hour and then turn the oven off in a couple of hours?" He set the timer for me so that I'd remember, kissed me good-bye and headed out to work.

So every half hour when the buzzer goes off, I leave what I am writing here at the computer, enter the fragrant aura of the kitchen, open the oven and remove the heavy lid to stir the ingredients in the big orange pot. A warm, fragrant cloud embraces me as the lid comes off. I am struck by the beauty contained in the pot. It is so pretty, this autumnal stew, so full of fall color, rich orange all dotted with dark raisins and bright yellow gradually cooking down into a lush, bubbling brown. Already in the pantry are the canned pears and figs of late Summer. Soon they will be joined by smaller jars of pumpkin jam.

I reset the timer and return to our sunlit study, throwing another log into the crackling flames in the wood-burning stove. The handle makes its predictable screech as I open and close the square black door. Buddha is curled up in her usual spot on the side table in the sitting area near the warmth of the stove. I realize suddenly that I am happy.

As I settle back into my wicker chair in front of the screen, I find myself musing about pumpkin jam. There is something about the combination of energies in that kitchen that pleases me greatly. The beauty, the aroma, the warmth on a cold day, the promise of comfort and good times in Winter, even the periodic interruption of the timer, a clear voice of order in the midst of rambling thoughts.

Then there is the mystery of the cooking process itself, rich alchemy of change, the letting go of one form, merging into another. And in the center of it all is Conrad's love adding the intangible ingredient that makes it all come alive. Peeling the pumpkins, stirring in lemons and raisins and apricots, turning on the heat and then entrusting me with the delicious task of checking up on it from time to time.

The ingredients are simple. Little more than pumpkins bubbling in a pot. It's love that makes it something splendid. Your love helps free me to see the beauty, to feel the warmth, to bask in the aroma, to respond to your invitation to pause in my search for meaning to help stir the pot.

Provisions for Winter. A warm place to call "home". Someone to love. Someone who loves me.

Simple pleasures. Profound gifts.

Jack-o-lanterns transformed into jam.

Thanksgiving Morning

IT IS A BRILLIANT FALL DAY. The cord of oak and madrone Conrad and I stacked together last month stands carefully ordered within easy reach of the back door, creating a rich pattern of alternating golden light and deep shadow. The whole house is filled with the aroma of free-range turkey baking in the kitchen, recalling many a holiday gathering in the past. In the middle of the table is an arrangement of acorn squash, pomegranates, persimmons, apples and oranges on a bed of Fall leaves in reds, browns and yellows. Conrad, his mother Vivian, our friend Diendo and I are sitting around the table cracking jokes and walnuts. The pantry is stocked with canned pears and figs from the trees in the garden and pumpkin jam Conrad made from the Halloween jack-o-lanterns. We are happy and blessed.

Conrad's loving companionship is a treasure that continually humbles and amazes me. We have fun, the two of us, and a lot of heart-to-heart time as well. The pleasure of owning our own home is proving to be a major blessing. I feel more settled than I have in years. This man and this home are strong anchors for me. He teaches me love through his simple acts of kindness. He is a caregiver and home builder of extraordinary competence.

We share a wealth of warmth, thoughtfulness, silliness, and grief as the AIDS epidemic continues to claim so many of our friends. We have learned much about acceptance and loving support, and have grown stronger as a couple and as a community because of the challenges we are facing together.

Together. I guess that's the word that most clearly says what these blessed days are about for me. We are all in this miracle called "Life" together; struggling, growing, learning to love, to give and receive, to show up and tell the truth, to remind each other why we continue to hope, to live.

It is as though we are all of us sitting around a great table offering each other nourishment and hope—our food, our stories, our tears and laughter. I sit here amazed by so much abundance, remembering all the things for which I am grateful, all the merciful ways in which life blesses us even in the midst of great pain and destruction.

To remember to claim all that is good. To grieve our many losses, yet be grateful for the precious time that we had with all that is gone. To allow the spirit once more to find its wings. To ponder the mystery that set life in motion and continues to sustain us. To focus the ever-active and often wayward mind on love, rather than ever-present fear. These are the challenges and blessings of Thanksgiving. To be reminded, to remember why we are here, why we go on loving.

I choose to be here. I choose to keep on. I choose to remember all my reasons for staying. I count my blessings; perhaps corny but true. I choose to continue, to go on loving and breathing, giving and receiving, struggling and arriving. For now, in this moment, I once more choose life. All too soon the choice may be out of my hands. Even now I am aware of a grace greater than myself. I join my will with the force of life that is everywhere evident and vibrant and strong. My choice is to be here.

Thank you, my friends for all that you give me, all that you teach me, the ways that you trust me, all that you share. Thank you for the music making, the shared meals and the laughter, and also for the tears. For letting me see what is most precious in you. Thank you for listening, for caring, for helping sustain me. Thank you for taking the time. Time so precious. Time so rare.

Thank you, Conrad, for this journey together, for showing me how to create a home, for teaching me to cherish the dailiness of living, for our many adventures out into the world and all the sweet returnings again to our own hearth. For the fires you've lit and the meals you've cooked and the quilts you've sewn and the faucets you've fixed. Thank you, my dear, for holding me close and letting yourself love again after Larry died. Thank you for saying, "I love you" as often as you do, for whispering "sweet dreams, Dear" before we doze off, for letting me hold you as slumber takes us away. Thank you for the way your eyes dance when I enter the room, for all the many ways that you care, for discovering with me the gifts in the plain and the simple.

Thank you, Mom and Dad, my cousins and aunts and brothers and your wives for accepting me even in my differences from you.

Thank you, Buddha my cat, for sharing your warmth with me and companioning my days.

Thank you, birds and butterflies, spiders and worms, zinnias and sunflowers, fruit trees and shade trees for creating a garden where I can sit.

Thank you, river, for flowing so close to my door, for your moods and changes offering me constant delight and adventure.

Thank you, my own sweet self, for not giving up.

Thank you, dear, troubled lungs, for giving me breath and letting me still sing.

Thank you, eyes that still see and ears that still hear, legs that yet carry me to the river and home, strong arms that still hug and soft lips that still kiss. Thank you, my heart, for still caring.

Thank you, Great Spirit, for creating me and setting me down in this place and time.

And thank you, sweet, long suffering Earth, for sustaining still this awesome, daily marvel of life.

All That I Need

You needn't bring me store-bought flowers
Bring me a leaf or twig or stone
Bring me the earth in a blade of grass
Bring me the sky in a fallen feather
Bring me the sea in a broken shell
Bring me a mountain or bring me a lake
Bring me a forest woven with song
Bring me your heart, no matter how troubled
Bring me your hand, let it rest here in mine
Bring me yourself, that's all I've ever needed—

Bring me yourself, that's all I need.

Loosening Labels

FOR OVER A MONTH NOW the cottonwood has been quietly shedding its golden crop of leaves. Except for the really wet mornings during our recent deluge, I have been spending time each weekday morning under its protection, reading a little from Jack Kornfield's book on meditation, *A Path With Heart*. Then setting the book aside, I sit for another half hour or so, with my legs crossed in the generous embrace of the Adirondack rocker, wrapped in John Sansoucy's white and black poncho which Charles gave me after John died. Most mornings the sun slants in warm under the overhanging boughs. The air is as crisp as a tart red apple, reminding me of brilliant Falls in New England.

Usually Buddha threads her way through the dewy grass to join me in my sheltering lap. She sleeps and dreams and shares her warmth with me. We comfort each other in stillness.

The leaves rustle over our heads with the least little breeze. I hear them let go. Now one. Now another. They slide down through the canopy and land gently on my head or shoulder or chest, like what I imagine angel kisses to be. They continue their tumbling descent to the ground, or settle into the space where my body meets Buddha's. She stirs and looks up with sleepy wonder. You can almost see her little mind reaching to understand the fall of the leaves. We are not under attack, she decides, tucking her cold nose back into the ball of warmth she's created, sometimes sighing as she lets go once more into acceptance and peace.

More and more leaves are letting go as the days grow shorter. They rain down together when a gust of real wind shakes the branches. Now, when I stir from my meditation and open my eyes, my lap is sometimes nearly full of glossy yellow hearts. Unless she's grown insulted by the falling leaves' overbearing attentions and jumped down from my lap, Buddha too is nearly covered with a blanket of gold.

When I look up I can see the sky dancing through the arabesque of branches. No longer a solid umbrella of green, the broken canopy embraces the air in a miracle of color and shifting forms. Vibrant blue filtered through golden yellow. The colors themselves contain healing for me, opening my eyes, my heart, the very cells of my being. They call upon me to stop and see. To open and receive. There is a mystery here which feeds me. I am like a famished man with old, cracked hands cradling a gift of bread. People and things for which I am grateful spill into my mind. My heart is like a window opening wide onto beauty. I am amazed and humbled by the good fortune of my life.

Life so precious. A tree to sit under. A sky to behold.

The labels I have worn to identify myself are one by one loosening and falling away. Like expanding garments billowing out from a body no longer constrained by belts and buckles, the names I have used to define myself are loosening their grip on my imagination. Some of my names have already slipped away. I no longer have need of resumes and credentials.

It is still tempting to cling to my labels: PWA (Person with AIDS), gay man, husband/lover, son, brother, recovered alcoholic, conscientious objector, landscape designer, gardener, writer, composer, singer, fund-raiser, friend, member of this and that support group, Californian, North American, Caucasian, male, middle-class, middle-aged, failure, success. They are the lenses through which I see myself and judge myself in relation to the world. It is tempting to wear these labels like some kind of armor (armor, amour—interesting connection). It is tempting to wrap them proudly and tightly around my fragility or display them belligerently, piteously, as merit badges and war medals demanding sympathy and respect.

But meditation and illness have both contributed to the loosening of labels. Both have slowed me down. Both have made me aware of the breath coming in and out of my body. Constriction and expansion are my constant teachers. Loss and limitation have become my allies.

Leaves are falling, falling all around me. They kiss my head, my eyes, my lips. Gently they knock against my chest, softly collect in my open hands. "Do you know who you really are?" they whisper. "Do you know who you *really* are?"

I am watching Death. Death is watching me. Kindly but steadily He poses a question. In a myriad of forms the question returns, again and again until I begin to hear it, to really listen and learn.

Wind gently teases the leaves to let go. As they slip down through the tracery of branches, I can see the sky more clearly. As the tree surrenders its rich robes of Summer, I begin to see the true form of the tree. I feel angels kissing me into awareness, gently tapping my shoulder, my head, my heart.

"Do you know who you really are?" they whisper. "Under all the various disguises you've worn, do you know, dear child, who you really are?"

Winter

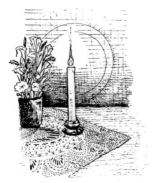

Silent Snow

SNOW IS FALLING. Soft, silent. I am in the sleepy college town in northeastern Oregon where my oldest brother lives with his family. Mother is at the retirement village here, alone now since Papa died last Winter. I am out for my morning walk in my brother's borrowed galoshes, Conrad's long johns snug under my jeans, knit cap pulled down around my ears, the wide collar of my jacket turned up against the cold.

I can see my breath as I ramble along, kicking my way through the fresh-fallen snow past stone walls and wood piles embroidered with white. Big, soft flakes land on my face like the "butterfly kisses" of fluttering eyelashes against my cheek that my mother used to give me as a child. I stick out my tongue to taste the snow, tilting my head back and standing still for a moment. I become aware of how hushed and quiet it is. No traffic, no people. Just the soft fall of snow. Silent. So silent.

I stand like a snowman in the middle of the walk, reflecting on the different kinds of silence I have known. There is the restless silence of abandoned houses where ghosts seem to whisper just under the level of our ability to hear. There is the dead silence that suddenly falls in a room when an unexpected and unwelcome key turns in the lock. There is the roaring silence of grief, the clumsy silence of embarrassment, the shocked silence that often follows the raw expression of anger, the devastating silence of unnamed shame.

There is the magical silence of children sleeping, the giggly silence of hide-and-seek, the windy silence of the Grand Canyon, Chaco Canyon, Canyon de Chelly, the profound silence of great cathedrals, Chartres, San Marcos, Notre Dame de Paris.

Then there are the sounds that come like jewels set down in the midst of silent space. The song of a bird on a frosty morning, the tinkle of a shop bell as you open the door, the whistle of a train in the far-off distance, the rumble of thunder before a storm, the mossy murmur of a stream in the ancient stillness of a redwood grove.

The most difficult silence to enter into has been the silence of my own heart. It is an elusive silence I chase in my meditations, never quite arriving in the place of peace I have sometimes touched. I patiently watch my mind's river of thoughts flow by while I sit detached and compassionate. I watch feelings surface, old memories replay. And as I watch, they all flow on. Sometimes for a minute or more, I am aware only of my breathing, my lungs quietly expanding and contracting, taking me down, down, deeper down. I start to drop into that deeper place I long to truly know. But I find after a time that I have once again wandered, and am thinking or planning or hearing or feeling. Gently I return to the breath, start to go down again, feel the peace. It is a cycle that repeats itself endlessly.

I am a novice meditator. It may take years of disciplined sitting to reach that place of inner peace. I may not have many more years. But I am deeply grateful for what peace I have found through sitting quietly in the garden or in the house or with other meditators. I am privileged to have tasted the great inner quiet.

Snow is falling. Silent, soft. A hushed, energized, peaceful kind of stillness descending all around me, settling within. Collecting on the rooftops, in the streets, on the lawns, making downy pillows of juniper and barberry. White birches and black elms cradle drifts of silent snow. Grey-blue spruce and dusky firs stand cloaked like snowy sentinels. Perfect little caps of white adorn the bright red fruit of crab apples and hawthorns, reminding me of clusters of round-faced children I've seen in pictures of Tibet, all bundled up and grinning happily before the camera. Silently it falls, like gentle understanding, smoothing away all that is ugly and raw.

I hold out my hands to catch the snow. In my palms the great downy flakes strike and hold for a brief second before they are melted and gone. Such brief little lives! Melted and gone. Silent lives. Born in silence. Fallen in silence. Part of a great white mystery of quietude I can't quite wrap my understanding around. How I would love to climb inside the silence of the snow! To be as still as a snowflake, as quiet and soft as a blanket of snow. To find that deep place inside of me where all the voices stop.

My inner cathedral.

Where only awe is left.

Baby

ZACHARY MICHAEL IS SIX WEEKS OLD. His weighty little head the size of a melon just fits in my hand as I gaze down at his swimming black eyes, his adorable button nose, his chubby apple cheeks and perfectly chiseled mouth with its astonishing repertoire of "oohs" and "ahs." He makes me laugh without meaning to. His tiny lips pucker at no apparent provocation, as if practicing kisses. His bald forehead furrows in a troubled-looking way, and then as quickly clears up again. Gas, I suppose. Suddenly he flashes a big, toothless grin, looking for all the world like the happy old Tibetan Sherpa whose picture so arrested me when first I saw it. I laugh out loud. I am utterly captivated by this precious little Buddha with his tiny hands not much bigger than my thumbnail and tinier fingers with toy fingernails. He grips my thumb, though, with extraordinary strength. His miniature toes are the tiniest of all, perfectly formed works of wonder attached to chubby little feet, chubby little calves, chubby little thighs and a doughy dimpled bottom. Baby, you are most wondrously made!

Zachary Michael is indiscriminate about who holds him. He gazes back at me without quite seeing me, I think. He doesn't quite have the focus thing down. It's more like I'm just another part of what's happening, or maybe not even what's happening, but rather what's *being*. The illusion of separation hasn't occurred to him yet. He gazes back with a level of trust and contentment astonishing to behold.

"He has no reason not to trust you," his young mother reflects as she sits relaxed and smiling while Papa prepares dinner at the gas stove nearby. I am sitting by the wood-burning stove in the comfort of their mobile home in the far-flung snowy reaches of northeastern Oregon, amazed at the trust this little guy is showing in the embrace of his bearded great-uncle he's never before seen. Just imagine: "No reason not to trust"!

Outside it is snowing. A gentle, steady snow of big, soft flakes. Inside is the miracle of a new family unfolding. Do they understand what a gift they have given me by letting me hold the baby? I have sat in support groups where other men with AIDS were denied the privilege of holding their own grandchildren. To hold a new life when your life is in jeopardy, to feel the weightiness of that little body, so full of promise, hope and trust. When were you ever that innocent and pure? Is it a place we can return to? Where do we go from here? How can I tell you what it means to one moving toward death to hold sweet life in its pure essence?

Zachary Michael is getting sleepy. His dark eyes are just barely open now as his heavy lids finally win the victory in the comic battle he's been waging, eyelids slowly fluttering open and then again as slowly descending, his big dark eyes swimming just off the coast of dreamland.

In his sleep he suddenly smiles the sweetest, most angelic smile. Then once again a cloud seems to pass across his brow. "Must be dreaming," I say out loud.

"What does he have to dream about?" Zachary's grand-mother, my sister-in-law wants to know.

"I don't know. Maybe he's dreaming about being born."

What are you dreaming about, Zachary Michael? What's going on in this heavy little head of yours? Maybe you're remembering where you came from. Maybe you still slip away to play with the cherubs. Why does your brow furrow and then clear? What is it exactly you're smiling about?

A story is told of a three-year-old girl whose parents had just made another baby.

"I want to be with the baby alone," she told her mother and father.

"But why, Sweetheart?"

"Just because."

They put her off, but she persisted. Then they remembered the intercom that connected their bedroom with the baby's.

"O.K., Angel. You can be with the baby alone now."

The little girl went in to see the baby while the parents rushed to their room to listen in. There was a long pause and then they heard their daughter say, "Baby, please remind me about God. I'm starting to forget."

Is there a God, Zachary? Is that where you came from? Is that where I'm going after I die? Have you lived before in other forms? Do you remember past lives? What could you tell us if we somehow could hear you?

Zachary Michael has a happy face, uncomplicated, open, nothing blocking the flow of love and trust and delight. I am struck by how much his open, round face and delighted smile is just like my mother's now that she's old. Now that she's finally laid down her crusade, given up her strong opinions and need to control, let go of her worries and judgements and finally found her way into safe harbor. It seems as though she has shed her skin and a sweet little girl has stepped out of the husk, trusting, vulnerable and dear.

Is it possible life is a circle, bringing us back to where we started? Does the striving and stress of midlife cause us to forget so much of who we really are? Does the slower pace of old age or illness somehow help us to find our way home?

Outside it is snowing. A gentle, steady snow of big, soft flakes. Inside is the miracle of a new family unfolding, a new life at its hub. Life renewing itself, the wheel of fate turning.

Zachary Michael's a marvel and I'm a proud uncle, gazing down onto his round, sleepy face.

Baby, please remind me about what truly matters, where we come from, where we're going, how to trust, how to love.

Baby, please remind me. Sometimes I forget.

Winter Wonderland

THE SNOW HAS JUST STOPPED. Across the white-blanketed landscape the sun is stretching a brilliant path of diamonds directly to where I am standing.

Despite my best efforts at searching the snowy landscape for serious and significant meanings, and despite my annual commitment to keep Christmas and all its hype at bay as long and as completely as possible, I find my mind insistently singing "Walking in a Winter Wonderland." It blithely plays over and over, like an old holiday record with only one cut.

I'm remembering every single word, and even though my inner critic is all puffed up with self-righteous disdain of how silly and trite this song is and how unthinkable it is for a Master of classical music to be caught associating with such tripe—nevertheless, I seem to be having a wonderful time. And the song shows no signs of going away.

"Why not accept it?" I suggest to my grumpy inner companion with a shrug. "After all, we *are* walking in a Winter wonderland. Just look at this. It's beautiful!"

Even the critic seems hard-pressed to deny the magic all around us. But getting in the last word, like the grinch who stole Christmas or old Scrooge himself, he pulls himself up, with rigid self-importance to his full majestic height and, head tilted back, eyebrows arched, pouty lips above set chin, threadbare overcoat clenched tightly about his regal throat, he says, "Hmph!" And turns on his heels, disappearing in an icy flash.

"Well, thank goodness he's gone!" I say to myself. "Now

maybe I can have some peace."

A flock of starlings wheels and settles into a nearby mountain ash tree hung with clusters of orange-red berries, each cluster mounded with snow. The birds start up in loud alarm as I resume my walk, and then settle down again as I get a few blocks further along my way.

How is it possible that each exquisite flake is individually fashioned, that no two snowflakes are ever the same? Seven inches of snow has fallen in the past two days, carpeting the land from here in eastern Oregon to Washington and Idaho, to Canada, Alaska and beyond. So much snow and no two flakes the same! The wonder of it!

How many billions of people are there? No two the same. Each one amazing. Each one precious. Some are healthy. Some are not. Some are brilliant. Others are slow. We come in a rainbow of colors and cultures, with different dreams, thoughts, foibles. We have most of us been wounded in different ways: hard ways, private ways, ways that warped and shaped and ennobled us. Our challenges have either awakened us to what really matters in life, or we have succumbed to a numb, troubled sleep as we try to avoid, deny or blame. We each experience our own story as personal, unique.

And so it is, although our lives are all related. So much diversity there is, and so many similarities. No two alike. No two separate. The range of human passions, interests and pursuits is staggering to me. Does the encyclopedia exist that captures the complete range of the human experience? It would be like trying to count up all the snowflakes in the world, while snow is still falling everywhere.

I am walking in the snow, aware and grateful that I can walk at all, see at all, hear at all. I am surrounded by beauty and love. How could I not want to sing?

"Sleigh bells ring. Are you list'nin'?"

About Jesus: Letter to a Friend

Dear F,

I hope you can forgive my long silence. It has taken me this long to have even a clue what to say in response to your note after we saw each other. A very big button got pushed for me when you asked if I'd consider letting Jesus into my life. It felt like you weren't respecting me for the spiritual path I feel I am on, in the same way I try to respect your path (although it makes me very nervous.). It felt like you were saying, unconsciously perhaps, "you're in trouble and need fixing. My way is The Way and I believe you'd be better off if you could let Jesus in."

I felt (not was, I know, but felt) betrayed. We have risked a lot with each other and have been able to respect our differences. I don't feel as safe now—although I still love you and believe we'll work this through.

I don't know that I know how to communicate what a loaded suggestion "would you consider letting Jesus into your life?" is to most gay people. I know you were extending it in love. I like a lot of Christians and believe most are good-hearted. But I am very bothered by what I see as the chauvinism of the dogma that says, "I am the Way, the Truth and the Light. No one comes to the Father except by me." That rules out a multitude of very fine, loving, compassionate and enlightened people—Jews, Buddhists, Sufis, nonbelievers, and creates (in the minds of the Christians, I think) a sometimes subtle and other times not-subtle-at-all belief that "we are better. We are saved.

You need help, reform, redemption." It is this mentality (which also exists in Islam, Zionism and other fundamentalist, chosen-people sects), I believe, that has fuelled many wars and hate crimes, and has allowed fear and hate and separation to grow to such awesome proportions in our country. Gay people are under severe and profound attack by the religious right. I do not mean to suggest that you are in any way linked to them, but I associate your suggestion with fundamentalism and it pushed a big button for me.

Thank you for hanging in there with me. I know I've overreacted but this is the best I can do for now. I'm sorry I don't have a better handle on these old hurts and current fears. Please forgive me for having been silent.

Still believing in us and wishing you well.

Love, Duncan

Candle in the Night

IT HAS ALWAYS AMAZED ME how much light is created by a single candle.

I remember the wonder and beauty of Christmas Eve as a child, where the flame from that single candle on the altar provided the light that gradually made its way into the farthest reaches of the darkened congregation. The flame was passed from hand to hand, candle to candle, until every face was ablaze with light. We softly sang "Silent Night, Holy Night" as the light grew ever stronger in our midst. I always felt the blessing of the glowing, flickering flames as my heart softened and melded together with the other souls opening all around me. We opened to the wonder of candlelit faces in the night and the promise contained in the birth of a baby born again and again, year after year, to light us through the bitter months of our doubts and fears.

I remember too the river of candlelight flowing down Market Street from the Castro after Harvey Milk and George Moscone were shot and killed, and several times since during annual AIDS vigils. We gathered in mourning before City Hall and took comfort in the light and our presence together. Like so many others, I left my candle burning at the feet of Abraham Lincoln. There was not a square inch left in front of him without a candle blazing against the night.

I imagine being surrounded by lots of candles when I go. I see myself lying in the midst of light. Not the harsh fluorescent light of a hospital room with the sound of strange feet and voices in the hallway. If it turns out that way, by some twist of fate, I will have yet another chance to practice acceptance. But if I could choose, I would go out surrounded by the soft, flickering light of a multitude of candles, each one like a friendly spirit guiding me through the night. Perhaps there will be soft music playing, or the sound of the ocean or the voice of a stream interwoven with bird song, or the low murmur of friends as they come and go. Or silence. There has never been quite enough silence.

Please don't call the coroner right away. The zip of the body bag is so brutally final. They say in some traditions that the spirit leaves in stages. And there may be friends who still need to say good-bye, even to a body that is no longer breathing. I would like to lie there for a day or two surrounded by the light even after I'm gone. If it is permitted by whatever powers guide the process on the other side, I myself may want to linger, to visit and contemplate, bow in spirit to you, my precious friends, and you, my dear body, that has held me so well.

I have never been to Mexico, but I have visions of the dead there surrounded by flickering lights. The spirits of the dead are not rushed away. They are allowed to linger, mingling with the living. I like that.

When John Sansoucy was dying, his Mexican landlady from next door came every day to see to his needs. She was a wizened old widow, always in black with a crucifix against her white throat. A woman of few words, she moved silently among us, removing soiled sheets and drenched T-shirts, returning a few hours later with fresh linens and, as likely as not, a bowl of hot soup. She moved with the quiet efficiency of someone who knew exactly what she was doing, what was required. I envied her her experience and her native traditions. I envied her her comfort and competence with the process of illness and death. I felt so awkward, trying to do the right thing, to be there for John when really I was there more for myself, a student of illness and dying.

When John died, the widow washed him and dressed him, and let his body rest before the authorities were called. She brought flowers in from their shared courtyard garden and kept candles burning in his room for a full week after his body was gone.

She and John had been neighbors in the best sense of that word. They had given each other the gift of their time and their stories. When we needed a picture for John's obituary the morning after he died, the old widow produced a smiling shot of him with outstretched arms on the beach, completely nude. "I've always loved this picture of John," she said, holding it up in the strong Spring light pouring in through the window. "Of course, you'd have to crop it here," she said practically, indicating the appropriate spot.

She stood in the sunlight, her white, gnarled hand nearly translucent against her black sleeve, holding the picture a long time while the little group of us who were there clustered close and gazed at this version of our friend, so whole, so happy, so totally unencumbered, with nothing separating his body from the sun-drenched air, the sand, the sea, the ocean of light stretching out all around him. The light seemed to permeate his very being, the drenching sunlight matched by his own inner sun, radiating out from an internal source flooding the molecules of air with joy. There was no trace of shadow in that jubilant smile, in those outstretched arms. There was no hint of the long years of suffering through addiction and recovery, no evidence of the exhausting brutal battles with personal demons and self-doubts, no indication of the war yet to come with the disease that would waste him and turn him old before his time. In that picture on that sunny beach there was only jubilation and utter freedom infused with light. Oh John, sweet John, my teacher, my friend.

Were the candles she lit for the living or the dead? In her mind, in her culture, is the line so distinctly drawn? I, among the living, was deeply comforted by the simple beauty and order she maintained throughout John's passing. The candlelight was especially important to me. It gentled me, helped me accept what was happening for John, for me, for all of us touched by this epidemic, by the ongoing challenges of life.

Perhaps it is the flickering, the subtle shifting of light and shadow, that feels so appropriate in times of transition. Boundaries are blurred. Straight edges curve. What seemed solid becomes liquid. Distinctions dissolve. Everything softens and wavers in the light.

Please light a candle for me when I go. For me, for my spirit, and for your own. In my own way, when I reach the other side, in whatever form it takes, I too will be lighting a candle for you. May its light join with the other lights that guide you. May the love we continue to share help sustain you. May you always remember how precious you are. Never underestimate the power of a single candle. Thank you for helping to light my way home.

To See the Wild Geese Fly

EVER SINCE FALL when I first heard about their migration over the Central Valley, I have wanted to see the wild geese fly. It became compelling to me, something I had to do, as important as the medications and herbs I take every day to stay alive. Vital soul work in the crucible of a body.

Right around the new year, thousands of geese flying south to winter in Mexico from their breeding grounds in Siberia and Alaska come to rest in the marshy bird sanctuaries just north of Sacramento. I longed to be there. All through the difficult months of November and December, I was sustained by the vision of a sky full of wild, honking beauty.

During December it rained relentlessly, knocking out power, closing roads and flooding people's homes and businesses with brown water and mud. New Year's Day was no exception. The new year came in cold and rainy. My heart sank. Yet another day for patience and projects inside. I had so hoped to be there on the first day of the new year. I longed for a powerful fresh beginning; renewed life and hope. I feared a slide toward despair.

The level of violence is so great in the world, the challenges so awesome that it is difficult to not despair, to keep faith with life and to claim hope in the midst of so much death and destruction.

"Always have something to look forward to." I wrote that on a piece of paper when still in early recovery from alcoholism. I put it, along with other things I wanted to remember, in a bright blue binder I called "My Resurrection Book," and left it where I would trip over it, to be reminded of what really matters when I was fumbling about in my distress and forgetfulness. It helped see me through many a dark night of the soul. I find it is still a valuable piece of advice. "Always have something to look forward to."

And so, all Winter long the vision of wild geese flying sustained me and drew me forward into a new year. This was my great hope: to see the wild geese fly!

As the rain came down relentlessly, day after day, I clung to the vision of the migration; the awesome pure grace, the powerful mystery of all those glorious creatures responding to the same deep necessity to lift into flight together at certain seasons and follow once more the compelling, ancient routes laid down by their ancestors. My imagination joined them up there in the sky, my wavering spirit finding strength in their company. With deep commitment we supported each other, flying in community through sunlit space toward a mysterious, sure and trusted destination.

Another week of rain came down with the new year and then still another. As one torrential day followed upon another, I began to lose heart. My dream started to dim. Perhaps it wasn't meant to be. Was this one more thing I would have to let go of? Yet another surrender?.

How long does the migration last? I wondered. Would I be strong enough next year if I missed it now? Would I even still be here this time next year? How could I have lived for forty-six years never having witnessed this wonder so close to home?

My hope faltered. The light behind the image of the great migration flickered but did not utterly fail. In my mind I conjured them one more time, sailing overhead in their long, shifting patterns, the sky full of wild honking, graceful, strong necks and powerful, wide wings.

Don't leave me, hope! Don't fly too soon!

I awaken this morning from waterlogged dreams to find sun streaming through the windows, the eaves still dripping after another night of pouring rain.

The kid me is already up and dancing with excitement. "Come on old man! Get up! Get up!" I throw back the covers, pull on some shorts and hurry to the back door to catch up with him, nearly tripping over the reclining cat. I excuse myself and step out onto the back porch, the cat following at my heels, into shirtsleeves weather, a glorious Spring day plunked down in the midst of a long, wet Winter.

Still damp around the edges, the sky is nevertheless undeniably and spectacularly blue. A few puffy white clouds, their fury spent, smile down innocently on a landscape teeming with color and light. The crows flap laughing from treetop to rooftop, calling and chattering, full of themselves, full of the day. I feel like laughing, myself, for the first time in weeks, like dancing crazy circles in the sun while robins and finches rapturously sing in the garden. The sun and the earth are at last reunited after the endless wash of tears. Brilliant, warm light pours like gold onto the steaming, receptive ground. The earth herself seems to be breathing, full and slow, in and out, exhaling her complex fragrances, acrid and sweet, from her deep alchemy of rot and ruin and resurrection. Moldering leaves and worm castings, fresh mint and sour grass, the dark humus of new soil being born out of the fallen glory of the old year. You can hear the ground percolating, little pops and rustlings as the breath of life finds its way down into the sodden soil.

Finally! It is perfect weather for an outing, our outing! The wild geese fly up into my mind with a great explosion of wings. I bounce back through the open door to announce to Conrad that "this is the day!" I find him in the kitchen already packing a simple picnic. He smiles over at me. I run to hug him. I love this man! Within minutes we pile into his trusty red truck and turn east through the rolling, green hills of Sonoma County.

Everywhere life is erupting with exuberance and sighs of relief. Baby lambs born during the cold, wet days wobble on new legs, frisking about under the embrace of this friendly gold warmth and light from a brilliant sky. Redwing blackbirds whistle and call on the rusty wire fences bordering the road. The lush fields vibrate with electric green that almost hurts the eyes, dusted here and there with great strokes of bright yellow mustard blooming early, breaking open the very heart of Winter.

This could so easily be Ireland or Scotland at the height of Spring. Amazing green! Amazing grass! Amazing grace! Like a chorus of hungry chicks when Mama arrives with a mouthful, the individual green blades seem to be shouting, bursting with uncontainable life force, a great, joyous clamoring, radiating energy in a swelling chorus up into the buzzing, vibrant air. The green grass of my soul shouts back in response and reaches tall, with the growing grass, towards the sky. Ah, if this were really Spring and not just a temporary reprieve. But Nature is not bound by human-made reckoning. It suits her fancy to be clothed in Spring today. Tomorrow she may return to her Winter wardrobe. But today, deliciously, gloriously, is Spring. You can almost hear Pan piping. Surely we will see him robust and gleeful, dancing among the goats around the next bend.

The patient cows, mud up to their knees, browse contentedly, oblivious to the exploding poetry all around them. They lift their heads from time to time from the grassy abundance and gaze off into the distance as though something in the hills were calling them. For a moment they strain to hear what seems to elude them. Their wild, unbred ancestors would surely have heard and responded to the great symphony of Spring that tumbles down the hillsides, bursting from the grasses, the stones, the oaks. It rolls across the meadows and fields and erupts beneath these cows here, tickling their stolid legs with music. Can't they hear the piper? Don't they feel the dance? They settle back into grazing. It is enough to taste the sweet grass and feel the good warmth on their broad backs and haunches. It is enough to graze and poop, dream half-formed dreams and lower their great, weighty bodies to rest awhile in the ooze of Spring.

For me, today, it is not enough. Not enough to sit silently soaking up the sun, to meditate and dream. There are times when a body needs to travel and see, to adventure, leaving the safety of home behind. Times when the soul yearns for pilgrimage. Today I have a mission—to see the wild geese fly.

Just up ahead, an early plum shimmers with white bloom before a stand of black, shady cypress by the side of the road, a study in contrast, like Mapplethorpe's photo of the bald black man and bald white man staring off in the same direction together. Like night and day, Winter and Spring, each lending meaning and context to its partner. Yes! Just so!

In an hour we have navigated the freeways between home and our destination and turned onto a rustic byway. This is flat farm country with only the rare tree. The fields are all flooded, blue sky and drifting white clouds fallen in the water, everything surreal and turned upside down. Water brims to the very edge of the road. We pass flooded businesses and old parked cars with water up past their wheel hubs. A road crew guides us across a treacherous stretch where water is spilling across the asphalt. Conrad gets a little nervous, thinking he sees water spilling from under the road as well. He imagines a road collapse and we are relieved to make it across. Just beyond the flooded section, a sign by the side of the road announces the entrance to the bird sanctuary. The side road disappears immediately beneath a brown lake. There is no bird sanctuary to be seen today. Not a goose in sight. Only a scattering of lone egrets stand knee-deep in water, watching our fools' progress across a waterscape even the waterfowl are, for the most part, avoiding. Where are the geese then? All flown south? Resting on higher ground? Have we come too late?

Our only option is to move forward, continue on into unknown territory, accepting the adventure on its own terms, complete with surprises and unforeseen detours. Scanning the sky for signs of life, we exchange benign glances with the fleecy clouds. They divulge no secrets. There is no sign of geese anywhere. Only blue space and white clouds above and below, extending for miles in every direction.

Gradually in the distance a great lone tree moves toward us, the only interruption in the flat, sodden landscape. Still bare with Winter, it looms ahead of us, stretching up and out into space. A giant old sycamore allowed to grow free, never butchered and pruned like its distant city cousins. The bare branches and stems seem to be hung with a huge crop of dark fruit. As we make our approach, the fruit starts to sing, exuberant and shrill. We pull up across the road from the huge, mottled trunk and its overarching branches and shut off the engine. Through the open windows spills the sound of a multitude of blackbirds, whoop-

ing and whistling, crowding the bare old winter frame-
work with wild movement and twittery song. The black,
feathered fruit assaults us with a deafening cacophony of
vibrant voices. In all this expanse of watery space, the
road has led us to The Tree of Life.

Rapt, we sit with windows rolled down, taking in the
great chorus of overlapping whistles and shrieks and war-
bles which dazzles the careful linear workings of my poor
brain. I surrender to the music, and let my mind be
washed clean by the sound. I let go of clinging to old goals
and visions, to problems solved and unsolved, to worries
and regrets. The past is past. Now, for this gift of wings
and wild welter of song, I am present.

How long have we sat here, merging with The Tree of
Life? When did my soul stop aching to see the wild geese,
and accept the magnificent gift of blackbirds instead?

The pilgrim's goal seldom unfolds in the ways she or he
expects. The fourth wise man never made it to Bethlehem—
he was too busy responding to life along the way, giving
away the jewels he'd been bringing to the Christ Child,
relieving suffering, offering comfort.

Eventually the road calls us on in a leisurely ramble
towards home. Adventuring together. That's the real gift.
The easy way Conrad and I have with each other. The
pleasure of good, comfortable company, enjoying the spirit
together in an unstructured and unpredictable day. It was
enough to be adventuring together. More than enough to
have sat timelessly under the singing Tree of Life. It was
enough. Now we were headed towards home, following
the road, meandering, dawdling. Turning left where another road offered, winding around in the watery dream
world.

Now, unexpectedly, we see the rainbow, a double rainbow actually, forming against dark clouds to the east. The

colors are just starting, arching up slowly from the soggy ground into the sky. Another gift! More to savor. A dark stand of trees perhaps three miles away is the only other thing on the horizon. As we continue south, the rainbow travels with us, approaching the stand of trees nearly due east of us now. Finally they join. My heart quickens with so much beauty. So much grace. The growing colors seem to be sprouting from the very center of the distant stand of trees. At this perfect point we pull over to the side of the road to take in the scene.

"Look!" Conrad is excitedly pointing at the rainbow.

"Well yes, I see the rainbow. That's why we stopped." I'm puzzled.

"No, no," he persists, a slight edge of impatience in his tone. "The snow geese!"

"Where?" I shout with excitement. Then I see them.

In thin white lines against the stormy dark sky the snow geese are flying directly through the beautiful arch of color upon color, the ancient symbol of promise and hope, modern symbol of diversity and community.

We fall silent with awe, taking turns with the binoculars. Flock follows endless flock through the sky. Just when we think we have seen the last of them and start to turn away, amazed at the majesty, grace and sheer numbers of what we've just witnessed, another thin line appears in the sky, followed by yet another and another.

I can almost feel the rush of wind from all those strong, magnificent wings and I long to be with them. My spirit flies up and joyfully I join them, honking and flapping my great white wings as I find my place in their formation and merging into air, we head towards home.

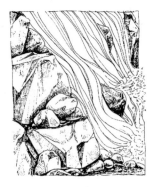

Spring

Lilacs

The daffodils have already come and gone
Early plum trees have given way to drifting white clouds
of pear and cherry blossoms scattered about town

We two together step out into sunshine after the long rain
Match our steps towards the river to sit over lattes
   at the outdoor cafe
To watch boats and seagulls, children and puppies

By a weathered old house along the way
Where a rooftop mockingbird sings every song he knows
An old purple lilac leaning over the walk, clamoring
   with bloom

Arrests us

And takes us back to parallel childhoods
On opposite coasts, longing toward a future
We haven't yet invented—to be here now—together, content

For a long moment with our noses buried in blossoms
We are barefoot boys still swimming in sweet lilac dreams,
Naked toes sinking down, down delicious into Spring mud.

First Day of Gardening

SPRING IS GATHERING MOMENTUM. Every day brings the return of some cherished member of the season—a fly buzzing, an iris blooming, the first butterfly, the first hummingbird, the first honeybee, the first bumblebee. This morning the fragrant blue iris that was always my mother's favorite and which I have transplanted into every garden I designed, has opened and is dancing gently in the morning breeze like a ballerina in tulle.

The cottonwood tree, so bare all Winter, is leafing out, bright yellow-green against the blue sky. It towers over the rest of the garden, coming back into its own. The dangly catkins are like fuzzy caterpillars suspended from the knobby twigs. Buddha and I have started meditating again out in the open air. Soon the green canopy will all be filled in and the heart-shaped leaves will start gently clapping again at the least little breeze. The plums have also leafed out and even have fruit already the size of my thumbnail. The fig too is fruiting, tiny hard little babies here and there among the budding leaves. Along with the airy yellow mustard, the fields and slopes are dotted with happy bright orange California poppies.

It is our second week of glorious, warm weather and our first day of earnest gardening. The ground has finally dried out enough to be workable. Conrad is rototilling the front yard where the little lawn used to be, preparing the way for the dry creekbed rock garden I have been planning, causing neighbors to crane their necks in curiosity, as we break from the tradition of predictable, neat lawns in front of every house. I had decided that the rock garden was more than I could manage, and wanted to let it go. But Conrad, no doubt thinking that I won't be around forever, said he *really* wanted a rock garden of my design out front. He would install it if I would design it and supervise the placement of the stone and plants. So now we're committed. It may take months, but we will have a stone garden and dry creek bed.

I am in the back, dressed in my long-sleeved denim shirt and long pants, and the Farmer John straw hat that Conrad bought me last year as protection from the sun. The drug I am taking to ward off another bout of Pneumocystis pneumonia, Septra, makes me particularly sensitive to skin cancer and other dangers from the sun, now that the ozone layer is being depleted. I refuse to give up all my pleasures, however, and work at weeding the perennial bed with my sleeves rolled up as I have for years. A ladybug lights on my sleeve, contemplative. Orange against work-shirt blue.

"Fly away home, Ms. Ladybug."

Being this close to the ground, I sense the earth moving as big worms and smaller worms emerge from the warm humus, poke around and over each other, in and out of the soil, stretch, contract; stretch, contract, movin' along in Spring.

I feel my fatigue start to take over. I find the sheltering dappled shade of the big cottonwood tree, overseer of the garden, and plop down exhausted in the Adirondack rocker. Before I know it I am nodding off, the buzzing of the flies and bees my music, the gentle breeze my companion.

Laundry Blessing

Conrad has brought in the laundry off the line,
Cold, Spring air infused in cotton
Holds a sunblown sheet to my nose and whispers "smell,"
Watches my eyes ignite, hears my "mm"
Then moves away smiling to fold and order.

In such small ways he blesses me.

Hope

I AM DRIVING THE FAMILIAR ROUTE to Berkeley. Here I lived and gardened happily off and on for nearly fifteen years, interrupted only by an occasional move back to the city to set up house with the latest, promising new lover. But Berkeley always drew me back after each failed romance, and I would return solo once again to the hills and gardens and carefully crafted homes of this historic town I love. For years I had longed for real community, to finally belong somewhere. As the years passed, my roots settled into the rich loam of Berkeley, forming a loving network of fascinating friends. I relished the cultural, racial and sexual diversity, the juxtaposition of intellectuals and street people. Berkeley made me think. I spent endless hours watching and writing in the ubiquitous cafes that line the streets, in the shadow of the great university. I formed wonderful friendships with enlightened and expansive souls, many of whom had, like me, struggled through years of addiction and recovery to emerge in midlife as healers. They work as psychics, poets, dancers, community organizers, teachers, gardeners, painters and writers. Mostly, they are women—Carolyn, Judy, Helen, Arisika, Jessica, Andrea and Gary. Many of my clients became my friends—Moneera, Sandra, Millie and Jonas, Ted, Lynda, Rita, Page, Jane. We would talk while I gardened. They often came to my concerts. I was invited in for tea. It was civilized, lovely.

It was hard to move away again. I stayed put in the

147

redwood shaded apartment in Helen's courtyard for nearly three years before taking up my roots one last time to be with Conrad in Petaluma. I have no regrets. It has been one of the best moves of my life.

Yet, I did not transplant easily to Petaluma. It took awhile to get a feel for the place, and one doesn't replace good friends overnight. It helped to find the cafe by the river. I love being able to walk there when I'm strong enough.

Berkeley still draws me. My old love of this university town by the bay, with its tradition of timbered Maybeck and Morgan architecture and lush English cottage gardens ignites once more as I turn east off Sixth Street onto Hearst. Even in this humble part of town, nearly everyone grows flowers in a pleasingly designed garden. Purple wisteria and white jasmine drip from the porches of modest two-story shake homes, as I drive along the familiar streets. Bearded iris in blues, purples and whites richly ornament the rambling front gardens like jewels gleaming in the beneficent embrace of the warm sun. Ornamental grasses in drier rock gardens, not unlike the ones I've designed and built here during the past ten years, catch the late morning light, becoming brilliant torches of luminous gold waving with every stir of air.

A few blocks up from Sixth Street on Hearst, I stop in front of the house numbered with the address I have been given over the phone. Generous, broad wooden steps ascend past tall flowering shrubs to the second floor front door and porch, where tattered and faded Tibetan prayer flags flutter in the warm morning breeze. A cat cleans herself in the nearby bay window, pausing for a moment to look at me with mild curiosity. My ring at the front door produces an immediate response by an energetic, bare-footed matron with tousled hair and an easy smile, comfortable sweat pants and an oversized sweater covering an ample, short body.

"Come in, come in. You must be Duncan."

"And you must be Jan."

She takes my hand and draws me into the sun-drenched living room where old overstuffed sofas and chairs in mint condition mingle with contemporary paintings and *objets d'art* in an environment at once sumptuous and homey.

"Just let me get my keys," Jan says, releasing my hand. In a moment she is ushering me through the art-rich livinggroom, down the back stairs and into a rambling garden. I feel a bit like Alice chasing the White Rabbit down a mysterious hole. Ducking under a rose bower trailing red blooms, we emerge once more into a pool of sunshine suffused on every side by lush green. As my eyes adjust to the sudden changes from shade to bright light, a charming studio room tucked at the back of the garden reveals itself, coming into focus like a dream come true. This is just what I imagined.

I shed my shoes by the door, beneath flowering vines tumbling from a low rustic roof, and I follow quick at the heels of my nimble, spry hostess as she pulls open the mullioned door. Visions of waistcoats, pocket watches and a blur of white fur still trail in my mind as I step through the looking glass into her magical domain. It is a perfect healing environment: hand-crafted redwood, mullioned windows banking both sides of the room and opening onto the garden where an old fig tree creates a dappled play of sunlight and shade through the windows. The room is alive and vibrant with positive, clean energy. Crystals, masks, handpainted prayers, twigs and cones adorn the walls and generous windowsills. Alongside the windows, two overstuffed chairs upholstered in old shades of rose sit in comfortable proximity with a little table in between. The rest of the room is given over to a bodywork table spread with white. It nestles in the long space obviously designed for it. We both plunk down in the overstuffed chairs while filtered patterns of sunlight and shade from the fig tree play across us both, weaving us into the fabric of the old chairs. We each draw one leg up under ourselves, the other leg trailing comfortably to the floor, our bodies turned toward each other across the little table.

I am immediately at home. I like Jan and how she lives. This is the Berkeley I know and love. Secret haunts at the back of gardens. The gardens themselves, half cultivated, mostly wild. Carolyn and her family created a studio and meditation space for her out of their old garage. Oak sprung floors, skylights, glass doors opening onto the garden. I have spent many profound and loving hours dancing and singing and speaking out my truth with her there. These women of Berkeley are quietly going about their explorations and healings in sacred spaces they have created in their gardens. You find them by word of mouth through a network of friends. You are quietly marked as one trusted. An invitation is extended. You arrive, remove your shoes and step across the threshold, stepping into sanctuary, into sacred time, into a circle of crones and wise women connected age upon age back into the mists of long ago. It is a privilege to be here.

I had been missing women's healing energy in my life. Neither my doctor, Tom, nor my acupuncturist, Bill, has been able to shake the wrenching, exhausting cough I have had since early December. Tom said there was nothing to be done, that the cough was the result of damage to the lungs from the Pneumocystis pneumonia of last year. But if that was true, why was it just showing up in December after a Summer and Fall of good recovery? It didn't make sense to me, certain that it was related to the long, wet Winter. I was not the only one suffering from such a long-term cough. I felt it was time to try a new healer—preferably a woman—so when Judy suggested Jan, I called her to make an appointment.

Now here we are, friendly strangers, with two hours to address my medical problems.

"First of all," she says with intensity, "you don't have to die of AIDS. That's a lot of bunk, a powerful myth nearly everyone's bought into. If you believe you'll die of AIDS, you will. But it doesn't have to be so. Living has a lot to do with how strong your will to live is." She stares intently at me. I look back mutely, feeling hope mixed with disbelief, aware of how much preparation I've already done for dying. Do I want to live if it proves to be an option? Could I make such a radical shift in gears?

"The most important thing you can do is urine therapy," she explains. "It has been around a long time and shows up in virtually every culture as a treatment for all sorts of ailments. There have been real results for many people with AIDS. What you need to do is drink a glass of your own urine each day, preferably in the morning."

Somehow, I feel no resistance to this woman and her assured pronouncements. She is extremely self-confident without being rigid. I'm open, taking it all in, like surrendering to a big wave in the ocean.

Jan is a dowser. She uses a little pendulum with a small lapis ball suspended from a fine gold chain with a turquoise stone at the bottom. The stone moves in a circle as she asks various questions of it. A strong "yes" response to her question causes the pendulum to circle more vigorously.

She douses a long list of food allergies to see what is

problematic for me. I am amazed at how fast she is working, going down the list quickly with her index finger, stopping only to double-check foods that the pendulum indicates as hard on my body. Only sugar, coffee, moldy cheeses (all of which I have already eliminated on my own), cantaloupe and strawberries (of all things, just when the strawberries are ripening in generous numbers in the garden!) seem to be problematic. Oh well. Something else to give up.

"This is great!" Jan says, looking over enthusiastically at me. "There are usually many more allergies than this. You're pretty healthy."

She proceeds to a list of healing modalities, checking to see which ones are best for me. Again, she moves quickly through the list. The pendulum indicates strong positive responses to urine therapy, Rosen body work, and talking to myself! When she gets to "writing" the pendulum goes wild, swinging vigorously in circles. Jan has no knowledge of my passion for writing, but the pendulum is clearly saying "Yes! Yes! Yes!" Jan looks over at me. "Well, I guess that's a yes."

"What's causing the cough?" I ask her.

She sets the pendulum in motion again, concentrating inward. "It's one of the drugs you're taking." I name off the half dozen medications I'm on. "It's the Septra," she says with certainty. "It's irritating your lungs." Septra is the preferred drug for preventing a recurrence of Pneumocystis pneumonia. I started it in November. "What alternatives are there?" she asks me.

"Dapsone and Pentamadine," I tell her.

She quickly douses. "Dapsone would be much better."

I'm not quite ready to request this change of my doctor based on one session with Jan. It would mean asking Tom to shift me from the preferred drug to the second choice for those who can't tolerate the Septra. "Why?" he'll ask. Will it be enough to say, "Because I believe it's irritating my lungs"? I'm certainly not ready to tell him I'm making decisions based on the advice of a woman with a pendulum in Berkeley. I don't want to run the risk of losing him altogether. Our relationship is already strained.

"You're also being affected by mold in your house," Jan continues. "Draw me a simple floor plan and I'll tell you where the problem is." The plan takes a minute to draw. "It's the bedroom closet, she says." Somehow, I already knew that. "Put a heater in there and turn it up high. Leave it for a couple of days and that should take care of it."

Jan seems to have answers for virtually everything. I'm a little bowled over.

"I can't find people's keys," she laughs. "My specialty seems to be medical questions."

What a relief, even if only half of what she says proves to be true, to have *answers*, real *answers* for a change! Tom seems, a good deal of the time, to be following hunches based on the information the endless tests give him. Often, he honestly tells me, "I don't know."

I'm feeling elated as our session continues. I feel hope. Maybe I really don't have to die of AIDS. What a concept! I'm not even just reading it in a book! There's actually a live person who seems very sure of herself saying she can help me.

"I usually charge $85 a session," she tells me when I ask about her rates, "but just pay me what you can. Or, if you like, don't pay me anything unless you find that I've helped you."

We've been together two hours. In addition to getting the information from dousing, she has also done some bodywork, concentrating on the area around the breast bone where the immune system, the heart and the grief

153

points are all connected. Finally we're complete for this session. We sit just looking at each other. A big smile breaks across my face and she responds with one of her own. We make another appointment, give each other a hug and step back through the looking glass, winding our way once more through the enchanted garden. I half expect to see the Mad Hatter and the tea party in full swing in a bowery corner of green.

Having said our good-byes I climb into my truck, excited and more than a little dazed. How does all of this fit in? What's really real? Am I dying of AIDS or just giving in to a pernicious myth most people believe in? Could I really stay alive? What would I do? Life after AIDS—what a strange idea! How do I integrate information diametrically opposed to what my doctor has been telling me? Do I have six to ten months left to live, or is there a whole new chapter in my life waiting to unfold if I play my cards right? To what extent does my will to live affect my ability to stay alive? To what extent are all the prayers coming my way keeping the positive life energy moving?

Lots of questions. For the real answers, only time can tell.

Time. That's what we're bargaining for here. More time. More life. But does it really matter how much time we have as long as we live fully while we're alive?

Too many questions. Opposing and seemingly equally valid perspectives. My mind is in knots.

Somehow I've driven the hour home to Petaluma without really noticing. What a day this has been! This is going to take a while to integrate.

Ah, sweet sleep, come and renew.

Ambivalence

IF I COULD CHOOSE BETWEEN LIVING AND DYING, which would it be?

That may seem like an easy decision to most, but the further into this process I get with Jan, the more I realize how conflicted I feel. Many of us, both sick and well, carry with us an ongoing ambivalence about being alive.

My friend Laurie teaches a class on death and dying at the local Junior College. She has her students do an exercise in which they make two lists, one containing all the reasons they want to stay alive and the second all the reasons they want to die. Every student, she tells me, has at least one reason they would choose dying. When I did the exercise two months ago with my therapist the "death list" was easy and long, while I really had to struggle to come up with reasons to stay alive.

I have invested ten years in getting comfortable with the idea that I would die of AIDS. It is not a bad path, to go out in the prime of life surrounded by loving friends and caregivers. In many cases, people are fascinated by this journey you are on, and eager to experience the process with you. Dying done well is a compelling focus both for caregiver and patient. We all have to die. To observe different deaths, some more or less conscious than others, is to learn important lessons about our own dying options when it comes to our turn.

There is ample opportunity these days, to observe and learn. So many friends have fallen to AIDS and cancer and other, more obscure diseases. For many of these friends it has been a profound journey. To be included in their process has been a revelation.

Now I wonder about what Jan is promoting—that I don't have to die of AIDS. I have been keeping my ears and eyes open for evidence of long-term survivors during this epidemic. But those I have been aware of, both locally and nationally, though some have survived for thirteen or fourteen years, their health eventually declined and now they are gone.

I *have* heard rumors of HIV positive persons with uncompromised immune systems who continue in good health, and I have heard of people who were HIV positive and are now purportedly HIV negative. If these stories are true and clinically documented, why aren't they front page news? Why aren't whole groups of HIV positive people converting to HIV negative status?

What I had not seen is any hard evidence of survivors. Until now. Now that I'm a hospice client on disability with ten T-cells recovering from my second opportunistic infection, I encounter evidence that some people may actually have recovered from AIDS. I've sent off today to Connecticut for the taped testimonials of prior AIDS patients who purportedly recovered to full health on the urine therapy that Jan is promoting. And I am in my first month of taking an experimental product derived from mother's milk being promoted by a doctor previously on the faculty of Harvard Medical School. He claims that after eighteen months on this product, all the currently-infected T-cells will have been replaced by healthy T-cells unaffected by the virus. And that the virus will be gone from the body entirely, the T-cells returning to normal range.

I don't know whether to invest time and energy pursuing these treatments or to think of them as hoaxes provoking misguided hope. I have decided I am willing to pursue these two alternatives, but nothing else.

I have had well-meaning but misguided suggestions offered to me from stinging myself repeatedly with live bees, to seeing a healer who, in a single session can eradicate all evidence of AIDS. I want to stop chasing around whenever someone claims they have found the cure. I want to sit still and let the peaceful, centered spirit take over my reality. If I heal physically, that would be fine, but I think it far more likely that my path is to learn Death's dance as I come closer and closer into Death's embrace.

Hospital

LATE-NIGHT FREEWAY SOUNDS of passing cars and trucks, the flash of lights, the hum of wheels. I am in the back of an ambulance being transferred from a little desert hospital near Yucca Valley to the nearest Kaiser facility in Los Angeles. It is after midnight. Lights whiz by outside. Until this afternoon when it became clear that my fever needed attention, I had been attending a silent meditation retreat.

"May you be happy. May you be peaceful. May you be free from suffering." I repeat this over and over to myself as the ambulance speeds along. I was just learning these phrases and letting their goodness sink into me at the retreat. Now they sustain me as I ride along. I am happy. I am peaceful. I am on an adventure. I am in the care of others. There is nothing for me to do.

After over an hour on the road, we arrive at a kind of loading dock where they raise the gurney and click the wheels in place. I'm whisked into the bright lights and incredible bustle of the emergency room of Kaiser Fontana, where they do an intake. I am transferred from the ambulance gurney to a hospital bed and helped off with my clothes and into one of those flimsy hospital gowns. Within the next half hour I meet more doctors and nurses than I can keep track of, and everyone has a string of questions for me. My main doctor is a soft-spoken, compassionate young Chinese woman who has recently completed her internship. I hope I'm in good hands.

Within an hour they transferred me to a bed in the

cardiac division, the only bed available. Today I was transferred here, to this small private room, its only window being in the door—presumably leading to the nurses' station. There is a nurse's call button, which I am pushing constantly. My body is like a waterfall. I am sweating so profusely there is no point in changing gowns. Pads, sheets, pillows and pillowcases are soaked through as soon as my body touches them. I was lying in a cold, wet gown on cold sheets with cold air flowing through the vents (State law). More optimal conditions for killing me with pneumonia could hardly have been arranged. I am growing desperate, standing up cold and wet next to the bed, pushing the button repeatedly.

"We *do* have other patients, you know," my nurse says as she flings open the door. "Please try to group your requests."

"But this is not O.K. I'm dripping, cold and wet—perfect conditions for the pneumonia we're trying to avoid!" This seems to get some action. She leaves me with a big stack of dry towels and blankets.

Some time later I am in a similar state. I have abandoned the soaked gown and am using anything I can get my hands on to dry off with. I've gone through the pile of towels the nurse had left me. Everything else is already soaked. I am standing there naked talking to myself when an East Indian in a three-piece suit comes in and leans against the wall observing my behavior. Finally he says, "I am Doctor Joshi, head of the Pulmonary Department. Please sit down." I ignore him, still searching for anything dry. The room is in total disarray. Finally I find a reasonably dry blanket and wrap up in it, sitting down to hear what he has to say.

I have been alone here now for two days, knowing nobody, trying to keep track of what is being done to me.

Thank God I have had the energy and intelligence to deal with this experience without advocacy. It *is* a bit lonely, though. I am pleased, however, to find myself lucid enough to ask the right questions and get action when action is called for. There are many too many drugs being dripped into me. I am being treated for Pneumocystis pneumonia, even though they don't know what I have. The Pentamadine drip for the PCP has totally destroyed the taste buds. Water tastes foul. Orange juice too—unrecognizable, metallic. The only relief to constant dry mouth seems to be ice chips. At least there's something. I smell to myself like dead meat.

I get to wondering if I'm not alone. I sense presences, like friendly guides helping me get though the day. I talk out loud and I sound smart to myself, even wise. I wonder if my spirit guides are about. There have been some moments of remarkable grace. I hear wind chimes—very sweet, light music and see what look like angel wings. Then I open my eyes, the music grows dim and I realize I am alone in the room.

Conrad finally arrives the third day. What a relief! Now I can relax. "May you be happy. May you be peaceful. May you be free from suffering."

It had been the fourth day of a ten-day silent sitting/walking meditation retreat in the high desert at Yucca Valley when I began spiking temperatures around 103 degrees. David Carr, who manages Jack Kornfeld's retreats, had arranged to get me a full scholarship and ride for this retreat. Not only was I enjoying much of what the setting and experience had to offer, but I had been hoping, along with David, that the higher, drier altitude might help ease the cough. With codeine cough syrup applications just prior to each sitting session, I was managing to sit through the forty-five minutes without disturbing anyone. When it came to the forty-five minute walking meditations outdoors, the cough was pronounced and I unintentionally drew attention to myself.

I enjoyed the walking. Foot-high cactus sported huge yellow blooms. Large pink primroses with grey foliage hugged the ground looking so much like the Mexican primrose we cultivate in our Northern California gardens, but here in the desert the blooms are twice as large. The tallest things around were the yuccas, most between six and eight feet tall.

Upon first viewing, the landscape seems bleak, but treasures lurk around every corner, all hugging the ground to avoid the wind.

It was very cold, and the wind cut through my poncho and blanket as I walked. In retrospect, I should not have been outdoors. There was a doctor participating in the retreat and he was asked to have a look at me. He insisted I be taken to the hospital right away, to determine why I was having the fevers.

Nine hours of testing and waiting at the local hospital revealed a dangerously low blood oxygen level, which was the determining factor in the decision to send me on to Kaiser Fontana. Franz, from the retreat staff, sat with me the whole time, and James Baraz, one of the retreat leaders, came and stayed with us after the evening Dharma session, remaining until the ambulance came.

Once again, I am having a steroid reaction. Both Conrad and the nurse note how compulsively I'm scribbling notes, trying not to miss any of the decisions and procedures. I'm losing sleep and my mind is working constantly. Yet the doctors insist that I need this drug. They've been in communication with my doctor in Santa Rosa and he agrees.

So we'll just have to put up with the lack of sleep and hyper energy.

They do a bronchoscopy to see if there is any evidence of PCP in the lungs, a procedure that involves running a tube down into my lungs. While they are at it, they also snip a sample of the tissue lining for culturing in their lab, looking for the possibility of MAC, another major opportunistic infection that shows many of the same symptoms as PCP: fevers, fatigue, night sweats. The tissue samples culture very slowly. It will be four to six weeks before they'll know if it is MAC.

But here's a good thing. For whatever reason, the chronic cough I have had since early December has stopped! I did shift from Septra to Dapson at Jan's suggestion, just a week ago. Then of course I am in a warmer, drier environment. I am on so many drugs right now, it is possible that something in the chemical soup has knocked out the cough. Whatever it is, I am relieved.

Finally on the fifth day, I am discharged. I feel great. Energized. It is a beautiful morning! I haven't seen the sun in four and a half days. It's wonderful to be outside again. I convince Conrad that I can drive and take over for him for several hours. Wildflowers grace the slopes next to the freeway. The bright orange of California poppies mixes with the purples and blues of lupins, an Impressionist painting.

We're headed home! I am elated. The steroids no doubt are exaggerating my responses, but the relief I feel is real— to be out of that little room, to be with Conrad, just us two again finally, going *home*. Home!

Resilience

IT IS SIX A.M. I had hoped to sleep until nine. I am in a hot bath, trying to counter the effects of profuse sweating that have plagued me since four. On my penis is a condom catheter with a little bulb on it right before it narrows to attach to the tube carrying the urine to the plastic bag reservoir. If you hold the condom up straight, it looks just like a little pagoda. It's fun. In the tub it collects water which you can squirt quite a ways. The kid in me is having a good time.

The condom catheter is a blessed addition to the repertoire. For weeks I've been having to wake every twenty to thirty minutes throughout the night, when the sudden urge assailed me. Usually I could make it to the pee bottle a few inches away in time. Not always.

Now, blessedly, save for the coughing and the night sweats which have been coming every morning by four, and occasional urgent diarrhea episodes, I can sleep much more soundly without having to respond constantly to the insistent urge to pee. In an average night, I pee a half gallon or more. Everyone agrees it's too much. No one seems to know what to do.

I have become a cough *connoisseur*. The cough that was with me for six months, since early December, was low, wrenching and exhausting. It was often productive, but boy, did it make me work for those little tokens of sticky phlegm. This current cough of the last few weeks is quite different, its central position being in the throat. Although its goal, too, seems to be expectoration, not much is there and nothing comes up. Between bouts of coughing, I listen to myself wheeze, relieved not to be actively coughing, making my already raw, sore throat even more painful. Sometimes there is a great gush of watery discharge. My nose drips, and I cough up loose, watery mucous. The call of the migrating geese comes to mind as I lie here listening to myself wheeze and gurgle.

It's a good thing I come from hardy stock and started out with a strong, robust body. I'm amazed at how many exhausting symptoms my body has been sustaining over the past month:

- night sweats
- violent, persistent coughing
- constant fever, ranging from between 99° to 104.3° almost daily
- sudden attacks of diarrhea which I do not always make to the bathroom in time, followed by a tiring, hour-long clean-up operation I'm not always strong enough to manage. Thank God for Conrad.
- interrupted sleep
- problematic appetite
- loss of 25 pounds since March (from 180 to 155)
- no T-4 immunity (last count: 10 T cells, a few weeks back).

One of the things that surprises me is that despite these daily challenges to my health, I continue to be resilient emotionally, spiritually, and even physically. Most days I have a number of energized and productive hours. I talk on the phone, I sit at the computer, I do a tiny bit of gardening.

I'm convinced that all the prayer energy coming my

way is making a difference, contributing significantly to this resilience I seem to have. Many people call or write and say, "I'm praying for you" or, "I'm sending you good energy." I know it makes a difference. Double-blind studies have been done in which one group of hospitalized patients received healing prayers while another group of patients did not. The prayed-for patients needed fewer medications and were able to leave the hospital sooner than those in the control group. *THAT,* I think, deserves our attention.

So I'm happy to have the energy I have, wherever it comes from.

This morning when I finish writing here, I am planning to practice my song-and-dance routine for the Talent/No Talent Show Conrad and his committee are producing for our local gay and lesbian association.

"You're going to do *what?*" Conrad looked at me incredulously this morning.

"I'm going to dance," I told him again straightforwardly.

He left the bedroom shaking his head. I've been rehearsing it all in my mind. With the show only a week away, I need to start practicing for real. My legs are pretty shaky and my voice a little wispy, but I think what I have planned will work out just fine.

I used to sing opera, art songs, and Broadway musicals, but no more. I'm hoping to resurrect enough of a legitimate voice to sing one last trio concert with Charlie and Sky at the United Methodist Church of Campbell, two hours south in the Santa Clara Valley, where I grew up. It was there I directed the five-choir program as my Conscientious Objector position right out of college during the Viet Nam War. I have another month and a half to get my voice back to sing that concert.

In the meantime, I have a breathy, sultry piano-bar

voice reminiscent of Marlene Dietrich. So I've decided to sing a torch song with the aid of a microphone and add a very simple dance routine while David Lisle plays an interlude. I've settled on Cole Porter's "You Do Something to Me." After the dance, I'll come back on the mike one more time and will mime Marlene, speaking to the audience in a French/German accent while walking to stage front. Settling on the edge of the stage, close and intimate with the audience, I'll sing her famous "Falling In Love Again"—but with slightly altered lyrics:

> *Falling off stage again*
> *Never wanted to*
> *What am I to do?*
> *Can't help it...*

Then I'll cry, "oops", and fall off the stage—about a two foot drop.

"You're going to do *what?*" Conrad asked for the second time. I think I can pull it off. It's good for a laugh.

You can't just lie around in bed all the time.

Garden Visit

I'M SHOCKED TO REALIZE how little I've been out to the garden lately. Everything seems such an effort, and I've been so exhausted. I've developed peripheral neuropathy in my feet and wrists, which makes it very painful to walk. Nevertheless, I have ventured out this little way today to see my old friends in the garden and here I am, sitting in the rocker under the cottonwood, listening to the gentle murmur of the leaves shifting in the breeze. Birds are calling, butterflies flitting and the bees are busy gathering up pollen. The air is so fresh and sweet.

The coreopsis and feverfew dominate the front of the garden with their sunny golden yellow and clean, cheerful white. Ripe strawberries are fragrant in the perfumed air. The little pink rose, "the Fairy", graces one corner of the path while across from it the mallow, like miniature pink hollyhocks, are coming into bloom. Cobalt blue lobelia with a white eye laces itself through the other plantings. Bachelors' button and blue salvia bring a bit of the sky down onto the ground. Swallowtail and monarch butterflies flit through like flying blooms. The little white and blue butterflies are utterly enchanting. Why have I denied myself these pleasures for so long? Had I forgotten how wonderful it is out here? The seed Conrad scattered is coming up beyond the perennials—zinnias, marigolds and sunflowers. They grow so fast, these sunflowers! Already they are waist high, like a little forest, green sturdy stalks and sun-dappled heart-shaped leaves. There is one that has come up at the front of the border in almost the exact location *my* sunflower grew last year. It will be interesting to see if this new sunflower and I have anything to say to each other.

Spring. Renewal. New life. Hope. It was a rough Winter. Just to finally have the rains stop has been a terrific relief to both psyche and body. So now it's Spring. I had expected to report on abundantly rich images and lively, unexpected blessings of the season. This was to have been the culminating season of the book, full of deep nature and humus, richly abundant with the secrets of Spring.

Truth is, most days my sense of outside glory is limited to the patch of blue sky and bit of tree I see over our neighbor's house from the bedroom. I am out of touch with the earth. It makes me sad and a little embarrassed to admit, but this is the honest truth of my year—not what I expected of Spring.

Day after day the verdant Spring gets lost for me in the shuffle of fatigue, night sweats and diarrhea attacks. Jamilla, the housekeeper from Hospice, is always making simple and beautiful bouquets which grace our bathroom and bedroom and bring the season inside. Spring has to come to me now. I can no longer rush out to greet it. I can no longer walk more than half a block before the pain of the neuropathy becomes unbearable. I go back to bed exhausted after each little venture out in the world. I'm missing a lot by being in bed so much of the time. I wish I were stronger and felt more intimately connected with the season. Nevertheless I am grateful for the sunny days, the songs of the birds (yes, even old laughing crow) and the patch of blue sky I see out my window. I am grateful for the jubilant Springs I have experienced over the years of growing up. It is, indeed, a miracle to behold the great, wet explosion of green out of the rich, new earth. And then the flowers follow in such abundance and variety, it staggers the imagination.

I sit here in the midst of Spring, happy that I made the effort to come out. My heart expands. I breathe in beauty, I breathe out gratitude. My heart reaches out to embrace family and neighbors. And still it grows larger, compassionately embracing millions of beings I've never met. There is something I hold in common with them, a certain consciousness of being, a certain spark, a certain hope. We are all points of light on the great living net. The expansion of heart at any point on the net enhances the whole, makes the whole grow brighter.

Thank you, butterflies and calling birds. Thank you, rustling trees and noisy crow. Thank you, Great Spirit, for allowing me another day on this incredible earth and helping me to see how I am surrounded at every turn by the precious and the beautiful and the healing.

Much Weaker

I DIDN'T REALIZE HOW WEAK I AM. This morning I went for my first solo walk in a month and a half, just around the block. It was almost too much. Conrad wrote in the log while I was gone, "I hope he makes it." He was on the look-out for me as I rounded the last corner toward home, moving very slowly, shuffling along like a tired old man. He had me take a cane with me, just in case, the first time I've carried one. I tried it out. Very seductive. Made walking a lot easier. But I don't want to become dependent on it unless I absolutely need it. I think I'll be stronger if I don't depend on canes and wheelchairs. If I'm exhausted, fine. But I don't want to make it a habit. So I carried the cane without using it. At least it let the motorists know I wasn't dawdling in the crosswalks just to annoy them.

Ironic that I was doing sitting and walking meditation a little over a month ago in Yucca Valley when I got sick and now I can barely make it around the block. The walking meditation took forty-five minutes. We did several each day. Before I went into the hospital, I had energy and health. After I came out of the hospital, I was almost too weak to shuffle around the block. Things change. You have to accept them and go with the flow. Otherwise you suffer needlessly, holding onto a past that no longer exists. I have had very little suffering, thank the gods! I'm basically along for the ride, not knowing what may be coming next, but able to find the good and acceptable in each new situation.

My spirit and mind are both strong and still full of plans and projects that assume the body's ability to respond. I push my limits, anxious to plant one more flower in the garden, making sure all the seedlings are cared for, watering things in. Gratefully, I usually have a couple of hours of reasonably good energy during the day so that I can get out into the garden or go for a walk.

I am reminded of Lois who worked as my gardening assistant in Berkeley. She had been bedridden after being nearly electrocuted in her previous job as an electrician. They gave her little hope of improvement. Her nervous system was fried. If she did heal, they told her, it would be a very long process and she must stay in bed and rest while the body tried to mend. Lois wasn't having it. She crawled out to her garden every day and poked about, planting, weeding, watering, steadily, slowly. It was her primary medicine and life-giving passion.

I'm a bit that way with our garden. I dig a hole. I sit and recover. I put a plant in the hole. I sit and recover. I water it in. I sit and recover. So it goes. Progress. The garden is already very pretty, blue and purple salvia mixed with lavender and cream-colored and pink yarrow as you first enter our little paradise. There is a pink rose in the center of the perennials, and in the background tall purple *verbena bonariensis*, pink and mauve mallows and a blue buddleia. Blue lobelia and cornflowers mix with yellow coreopsis and white feverfew. Beyond the perennials the sunflowers, zinnias and marigolds are growing, a blaze of hot colors later in the season. Across from the hot colors we've dug a new broad bed for a blue and purple buddleia collection to cool the eye after all that fire, and to give all the butterflies a treat.

I am grateful for what energy I have. Grateful that I can still dig a hole, plant a flower. Grateful to sit in front of this screen and make words that print upon the page.

Everything is so much slower now, but as long as I can do a little something each day, I am content.

Acceptance

I'M PRETTY MUCH O.K. if I'm sitting or lying down. It's getting from one place to another without help that can be hazardous. Even though I consciously make the transitions slowly, I have been passing out, or nearly so, clinging to furniture and walls, waiting while I recover or go over the edge into a fall.

I was lying in bed this morning thinking of things I had to be grateful for. "No diarrhea for a whole week!" I'm thinking. I've been awake since three A.M., just like yesterday morning, only without the chills and teeth-chattering that drove me out of bed and into a comforting hot bath. My fever was 100 degrees getting into the bath, 104 degrees by the time I got out. I can't run the bath as hot as I'm used to, Conrad tells me, and can't stay in for as long, if it's going to make my fever shoot up that dramatically. I need to keep careful tabs on my temperature while I am in the tub, and get out before it becomes problematic.

At bedtime last night I had my first normal temperature for weeks—98.7.

I shouldn't have driven to the acupuncturist this morning. Misjudged the parking space in the lot and crashed into the garbage bin. A lot of effort to get up the steps. Moving very slow. Slowly shuffled across the room to an available chair and collapsed. Gail and Trish recognized my condition and were so kind. I may not be able to come in for awhile if I'm not stronger than this. Conrad wants me to give up driving for now. I guess he's right. The weakness affects my thinking and judgement as well as my physical capabilities. My acupuncturist says he'll come visit me at home from now on.

More change, adjustments. More need for acceptance. I've been keeping up pretty well. But no driving? That's going to change things considerably. It means I can't go to my favorite group on Thursday nights. It is an AIDS support group at the Center for Attitudinal Healing in Sausalito, forty-five minutes south of here. That's a hard one to let go of. It means a lot to me. But when I hold on, I find I suffer. I pray for acceptance.

As soon as I shift my focus to what is, and start to let that reality take over my consciousness, I just naturally settle into this new way of being. Although this new way involves loss and limitation, I still have a choice as to where I place my focus. And within the smaller frame imposed by the new limitation, the lens of the eye and the soul adjusts to a closer, more intimate focus.

There is a wonderful activity we used to do with the children at summer camp, in which we gave each camper a piece of paper with a square inch cut out of the center. They lay the paper down on the grass and watched the activity within the square. It was always astonishing to them what they discovered, how much that square inch teemed with activity.

Closer focus. Great surprises.

There is a woman I've heard of who is quadriplegic and confined to her small inner-city apartment. Every day for months a young man has delivered meals to her. Finally one day his curiosity got the better of him and he blurted out, "How can you stand this? What keeps you going?"

"Oh," she said, smiling over at him, "see the brick wall

outside my window? Every afternoon the sun moves slowly across that wall. It is the most beautiful thing! I wouldn't miss that for the world!"

From such teachers I learn grace.

House of Cards

CONRAD COMES INTO THE BEDROOM this morning and kneels down by the bed. "I just need to tell you I'm not ready for you to go," he says. "I want more time with you."

I've been talking about wanting to leave by Fall. "How much time would you like?" I ask practically.

"Thirty or forty years—but at least another year."

"But that means going through another Winter," I protest.

"Winter is harder on me than it is on you!" he responds with fervor. It's true. He can't stand the cold. He starts dreading Winter when Summer is at its warmest and most luxuriant, when it seems thoughts of Winter would be nowhere to be found.

"I'll try, honey," I say somewhat skeptically. To myself I think, "It would be lovely to see another Spring. I think I could do it."

I'd be doing it for Conrad, though. *I'm* ready to go *now* and I really would rather not experience another Winter, especially if it is as relentlessly wet and cold as this past one. That's highly unlikely, of course, given California's pattern of a wet year being followed by several dry ones. Johnna, my Hospice nurse, says it's my death and I get to decide when I want to go. That as much as I love Conrad, I need to do what's right for me.

But I appreciate Conrad's request. He told Larry that if it was at all possible, he wanted Larry to die in his arms.

And Larry did. It doesn't hurt to ask for what you want.

Conrad is scared. He's really not ready for this. I feel him pulling back, protecting himself, creating distance. This hurts. He becomes extremely busy, working long hours to cover his anxiety, I think. His face is strained much of the time and he spends time away with friends. Actually, I heartily approve of this last strategy. Not to get away, as most everybody knows, is a pretty simple recipe for burnout.

Well, we'll just have to see how much control I can exercise over the scheduling of my demise. I can't really tell when this weakening house of cards will finally come crashing down.

T-Cells

JOHNNA CALLED THIS MORNING to give me the results of my latest blood work. She was concerned that I would be upset, and approached the subject with her usual sensitivity and concern. After carefully talking around it a bit, she finally told me.

0 T-4 cells.

I laughed, relieved, I think, at the clarity of the message and the gift of being able to relax into the perspective that my body is headed toward physical dissolution.

"I didn't get to name them!" I complained playfully to her. "When they got to seven, I was going to name them after the seven dwarfs."

One of the hardest aspects of the journey this past year has been the balancing act required to keep my mind and heart open to the opposing perspectives that I am gradually dying, and that I can survive. I am relieved to finally lay down that nebulous, elusive possibility of survival and embrace once more the process of dying.

I believe the life-affirming work I have done has greatly enriched my life, but that it has not been enough to reverse the direction of this disease in my body.

Jan would challenge me not to take this lab work too seriously, certainly not as an indicator that death is, after all, the destination of my journey. But I have juggled these opposing perspectives long enough. I have grown weary trying to feed energy to a survival vision that feels increasingly difficult to sustain. It has been a fascinating side journey and taught me important lessons about my ambivalence in living, and about the powers that are available to us all if we can but tap into them. It has been my first experience with a powerful alternative healer. I have loved it. And I love her. I wish I had met Jan years ago while I was still just HIV positive. I suspect our work together may have had a stronger impact on my body then. Yet it feels like we met when we were meant to— toward the end, and that perhaps her greatest contribution has been to introduce me to my Spirit Guides and the higher, more subtle vibrational realms in which they dwell.

It is a relief to return to the path I have perceived myself to be on for the past ten years: the acceptance and anticipation of death, sweet death, mysterious death, transition to something finer. I have had intimations of angels and clouds of love-filled light in my sick room. I have felt surrounded by spirits who care for me. They seem most strongly present when I am most challenged physically, and when my mind loosens its grip on what it takes to be concrete reality and allows itself to float. I look forward to revisiting that place of angels and dwelling there more constantly, opening more and more to glory and peace.

So T-4 cells, thank you for your long, valiant struggle. You have finally been able to lay down your campaign. You are finally able to stop.

Oh, Dear Body

I WAS NAKED IN THE BEDROOM this evening, and was shocked to see in the full-length mirror how thin you've become.

Little more than a year ago, you were a robust Scotsman of two hundred ten pounds, easily able to handle fourteen tons of stone to terrace a hillside garden. You lifted each stone at least four or five times, trying this one with that one until you found the fit.

Nothing I'd rather have been doing. Like a boy playing inside a strong man's body, taking pleasure in physical strength, sensing his connection with a long tradition of stonebuilding, slowly working a huge, satisfying puzzle. I was being paid well to be engrossed in what I loved best about gardening: the placing of stones. Sometimes I fancied I could hear them singing, vibrating slowly inside their whirling environment of electrons and neutrons, seemingly so solid, so dense, and yet filled with spacious spinning. I felt their history, their earthiness, how long it had taken to build the beautiful lichen colonies in sea-green and bright yellow.

We were going to put in one of "my" stone gardens out in the front yard. Even rototilled and prepared the soil. One afternoon, Johnna and I sat out on the sidewalk in white plastic chairs and directed Conrad's efforts as he contoured the earth, making two levels with the suggestion of a dry waterfall. And then this Spring, with illness and exhaustion week after week, I have not been up to

even thinking about it. Conrad could sense my waning
interest in the project.

"I really want the front garden to be one of your rock
gardens. When I come home, it will be like coming home
to you," he said one day. "If you could just design it, I can
install it."

"Yes, of course, I'll do what I can."

Now you're weighing in at one fifty-five—that's fifty
five pounds of muscle gone during the past year. The
weight seems to take a slide periodically and then stabi-
lizes at a new weight. For a long time it was one-eighty.
Now for awhile it's been one fifty-five.

You're like an old man with sagging skin where muscles used to be. My mind can't keep from returning to the
images of the shocking, naked old people in the "medical
evaluation" scene in Stephen Spielberg's heart-rending
movie "Schindler's List." Old men and women are forced
to run around the courtyard in a circle, naked, to prove to
the Nazi authorities that they still have enough health and
vitality to be of physical use to the compound. The weak
ones are singled out to be shipped away.

Oh, poor body, you're starting to look like that. The
proud firm butt, the muscular thighs, the broad proud
chest, the full lips and cheeks — all changing from day to
day, sagging and dwindling away. You have always carried
me so well, I've taken you too much for granted. Now I
can barely get out of bed some days. I should have realized
a long time ago that with no exercise the leg muscles
would atrophy. Finally, this week, I took action and joined
a gym. I got around well with my walker and made use of
the pool where I swam several laps. That was three days
ago. In the past two days I haven't been able to trust
myself to stay on my feet. I seem much weaker. My knees

keep buckling. I'll need to get stronger before I can go back. Hopefully, I can get enough exercise to rebuild some of the muscles in the thighs. The calves, fortunately, are still strong.

We are like old intimate friends, you and I, sweet body. One of us is gaining momentum and enthusiasm. The other may rally, but has been severely challenged and is in decline. We're like old lovers who know each other so well and love each other so much that another wrinkle, a slower pace, a sagging body part are all acceptable. They are even lovable changes, because they're part of the beloved's body.

I love you, body. I love the way your fingers unfold in the morning light, as if of their own accord, not yet engaged in any projects. I love your eyes that look back at me in the mirror with nothing to hide, no unresolved shame. Beautiful eyes, sometimes blue, sometimes green—green like the ocean, sparkling with light.

I love sleeping with you every day, feeling myself slip deeper down inside you. I feel leg upon leg, bone upon bone, sometimes painfully as I try to get comfortable on my side. Ah, then finding a position that works for you, for me—what a good moment that is! I love breathing in the sweet scent of the pillows, stretching a long arm across the bed, letting my fingers gently trace the edge of the furthest pillow. I like being long. I like being tall. I may no longer have a big strong body to take pride in, but I still like to feel myself stretch out inside you, body, to fill up the spaces you offer me to live in.

We've been a good team for all these years. We're a good team still.

Chinese Puzzle

WHEN PEOPLE ASK ME HOW I AM, I respond with my physical, emotional and spiritual conditions. It almost seems that the weaker I am physically, the stronger I am spiritually. There is an opening to the spiritual realm that seems to come with depleted physical resources. Gratefully, I have been remarkably stable emotionally, usually in good humor, occasionally impatient with lack of energy if it goes on for more than a day or two. But generally I have a lot of acceptance.

It is like living a life within a life, a disease inside a body inside a personality inside a spirit inside a soul. Like those intricate carved ivory balls cradled inside one another, each holding the next in size, from large to small. Have you seen them in Chinatown? Like so much of what the Chinese mind and artistry have produced for centuries, they astonish me and tease my brain. How did they do it? How is it humanly possible? And having achieved such beauty and perfection of detail, what does it mean, this independently rotating ball trapped within a ball within a ball within a ball? For us, perhaps soul is the very center, and then spirit, and then body.

I remember the Chinese puzzle box my grandmother gave me when I was young. You had to navigate a series of secret sliding wooden panels, each unlocking the next, until at last the inner sanctum became open and free—the hidden center where your treasure was stored.

The gradual disassembly of physical strength, sliding the panels away, seems to open to the inner sanctum.

Visitors

DRIFTING OFF TO SLEEP these past several nights, beings present themselves to me, sometimes singly, sometimes in groups. I am the invalid. They are the visitors. They gather congenially about my bed. We ramble along in pleasant conversation and I feel surrounded by goodness and light. I am actually speaking out loud and I hear their voices as strong as my own. Moved by the love I feel coming from these radiant beings, I reach for their hands and feel only air. I open my eyes. No one is there.

Be Still and Know

LAST NIGHT DRIFTING OFF, my mind was rambling along, thanking and invoking and praying and watching my breath. Suddenly I noticed dim, white, ghostly forms, like glow worms swimming in rather chaotic but energetic circles against a black ascending space. A voice coming, it seemed from inside the black center said,

"Be still, and know that I am God."

My mind chatter stopped and for several minutes I basked in this strange light with my arms raised from their elbows, palms open, a natural gesture of praise and receptivity that is common in several religions to which I've been exposed.

"Be still, and know that I am God." The one I'd come seeking. The one that was now speaking, bidding me to be still, stop all the effort and motion, just lie where I was so that my quiet, receptive body, mind, and spirit could receive the invited, ultimate guest.

"Be still. Stop doing. Stop writing. Pay attention. Observe. Allow me to introduce myself."

"Know."

"Let us be intimate. Experience me through all your levels of being."

"That"

"I Am God."

"Welcome!"

"Be still."

"Pull up a chair."

"Be still."
    "Is there anything I can get for you?"
"Yes. Silence."
    "You got it."
"No. You just did."

The Man Who Burned Up While Surrounded by Blue

IT HAPPENED SEVERAL YEARS AGO NOW, but it's a story worth telling. It comes back to me whenever I see blue daisies, *felicia ameloides*. This morning a friend brought a pot of them for me, that are now sitting by the computer. Such a beautiful color. My mother's favorite, and mine.

I never asked his name. Once I finally noticed him, his delight at having caught my attention seemed to make names irrelevant. I was installing a tiny backyard garden in San Francisco during the early years of the epidemic, and my early years of recovery from alcoholism.

I think it was the first time in recovery that I actually saw the sky. One of the effects of addiction for me had been that I was aware of only dark shapes and blackness. I was almost always in a state bordering on panic. The sky, birdsong, sunshine had all disappeared from my consciousness.

The man who burned up while surrounded by blue had to work hard to gain my attention as I placed brick next to brick, my self-obsessed thoughts rambling around in their gloomy maze trying to find the way out.

Several mornings now, when I'd come to work, I'd find a sky-blue daisy with a bright yellow eye staring up at me from the most recent bricks I'd set. In half-consciousness I'd brush it away, wondering how they'd gotten there, but not being aware enough to give it my attention.

Finally, one morning I couldn't miss what was happening, as yet another blue flower fell, like a wayward piece of sky, directly in front of where I was crouched in concentration. I looked up to the tiny deck of the second-floor flat to see that there was a wine barrel full of blue daisies, and above it a blue-eyed laughing man with blazing gold hair. And the blue sky. I realized I had not seen the sky in years. Blue upon blue upon blue surrounded by laughter and light.

"I thought you'd never look up," he smiled down on me.

"I'm sorry," I fumbled, slowly coming to speech, as if swimming through murky confusion to be dazed by the sudden and brilliant transition from black depths to light. I was dazzled, and not a little charmed by this blithe spirit full of light and mirth. The striking blue color and the enthusiasm of this fellow was enough to lighten me up a little.

After that morning, I started looking for the blue daisies. They were always there. When they weren't, I could count on one to come drifting down and a radiant face to greet me as I looked up into those blue, blue eyes and the expanse of blue sky behind him. Gradually we got to know each other a little. He was a fine porcelain maker. It was his passion. He had volunteered at Project Inform for years but was now too sick with AIDS-related opportunistic infections to get out much anymore.

One morning when I came to work, he was waiting for me. He wore rubber overalls tied at the ankles and was covered from head to toe with porcelain dust. He looked like a very animated ghost.

"Come up! Come up!" he insisted. I had never seen anyone so highly charged before. He was practically jumping out of his skin. I dropped my tools and made the easy ascent to his deck. "I've finished!" he exclaimed, with a sweeping gesture that took in both dining room and kitchen. There was indeed a beautiful collection of vases displayed on the diningroom table and the kitchen counters. White porcelain dust completely blanketed the two rooms and their contents as I rambled through and appreciated the subtle differences between vases that, at first glance, had seemed identical.

"I was up all night and I'm finished! My life work finally complete before I go!!!"

His face actually radiated light with such intensity it was difficult to distinguish any of the features, except for the blazing blue eyes. I would not have been surprised if he had burst into flame. He explained the rubber pants and their ankle ties. "I couldn't be bothered to stop for the diarrhea."

"And here's the best part," he told me with tears in his eyes. "My father has agreed to have the collection bronzed. I have never asked him for anything before as an adult. We haven't been close but I've always wanted a one-man show of my work. Seeing them bronzed has been my greatest dream, but it was always too expensive. Now my father has finally come through for me! How could anyone possibly be happier than I am!

"The vases are beautiful" I told him. "I'm glad you were able to finish them."

"Thank you," he said, the fire banked a bit. "I think I'll rest now."

He shuffled towards the bedroom.

The next day when I came, I looked for my blue daisy. There was none. I went upstairs to peek in the window. All the white, dusty furniture had been pushed to one side of the room. I sat on the top stair, musing sadly to myself and leaned up against the old gray railing post.

He was gone.

He did what he wanted to do. At the end, he held nothing back. He left in a conflagration of pure fiery spirit.

I missed him as my work progressed—his ebullience, his hope, his passion. I kept thinking of the blazing blond hair like a halo about his face and those piercing blue eyes with life brimming from their laughing edges.

In the Spring, grape hyacinths I hadn't planted started coming up everywhere. Sky blue hyacinths bordering the brick patio, following the ascent and descent of the stairs. I looked up into the blue sky. I thought I heard laughter, like bells tinkling far away in the wind. Didn't I just catch a glimpse of blue eyes blazing?

Live 'Til You Die

"LIVE 'TIL YOU DIE." Have I done that? Is it enough? Can I push away from the computer now, trusting that the journey I've recounted may have meaning for some of you out there who are still going on? The finish line is very close for me. I think I'll have just enough energy to cross over. It is a statement of exhaustion and completion.

I remember my father, such a good, involved man, uncharacteristically asking one day in his early eighties, "When do I get to rest? Haven't I earned some time in a rocking chair?" His frustration was palpable. He was trying to detach from a lifetime of service and involvement. Rest was suspect in the culture which raised him, a luxury one could ill afford even at age 87. His last years were spent in quiet rebellion, sitting in front of the TV, sometimes dozing, sometimes with his hearing aids turned off. Yet the day before he died, he was leading the exercise class down the hall from where he and mother lived. He loved people. He was a natural leader.

At 90, Ruth Whitcomb, a long-time friend and gardening companion who lived in a little seaside cottage in Carmel, when I asked her what her years had taught her and what she might have to say to someone with a life-threatening illness, told me with no hesitation,

"Be yourself. Learn to say No, but don't be afraid to say Yes. Be willing to make mistakes. Most importantly, live 'til you die!"

It's been a good long run, and this last year, at a dramatically slower pace, has been a joy, a challenge and revelation. I am ready to go at any time. I have lived a good, full life.

It is a redeemed life, a salvaged life, a life that quite nearly was in the gutter, but thanks to the help of many it got turned around. I feel like an inmate in a big hospital with lovely grounds where I have been wandering through the tall, dark garden maze, and have found my way through. I am resting now on a bench in the sun, against an old stone wall, waiting for the white-clad attendants to come for me.

Accepting death is not a popularly supported position in this culture. I feel the pressure of friends who expect me to hold on, to keep fighting, to still believe in miracles. They're not ready to let me go. Shocked by my decline, many had looked to me to be the exception, as I had been in such good health for nearly ten years.

Some are jealous that I get to leave, that I have a way out. They wistfully look toward their own futures with a mixture of hope and dread.

But acceptance comes one day at a time, I've learned. Moment by moment.

The seasons are turning. Soon it will be time to be going.

Knowing you were here has helped sustain me, given me passion and purpose. Thank you for the years, for the moments we have shared.

Cherish one another. Take time to pet the cat, and look up to see the sky.

May you keep hope alive.

Go well, gentle spirits. Live 'til you die.

J Am Worn Down

I AM WORN DOWN, a smooth stone in a stream bed. Sun dappled, wet and tumbled, one among many. I had thought to be the mountain, majestic, viewed from miles around, a place for pilgrimages and the dispensing of wisdom.

My wisdom is in resting here and feeling the water about my bones.

I did not go peacefully down the mountain. I did not approve. I did not agree. I did not understand how I was being shaped. Overwhelmed by blinding torrents, I crashed down gullies, lodged in crannies against twisted roots, tried to dig in, tried to hide. I tumbled brutally against other stones. We believed in the myth that we were contenders. We jockeyed for place, desperately competing to hold our grip on the mountain.

Sometimes I'd come to rest for awhile. The current would toss me off to the side. I'd look around to get my bearings, catch my breath and start to adjust. Sometimes I even got comfortable, totally forgot my dream of the mountain. I'd start to settle, find my place, accept my fate, turn away from the mountain altogether. Or so I thought.

We may not be able to remember our dreams, but that doesn't mean we don't have them. The mountain is a dream that won't go away. Even in my deepest sleep the dream festered and grew, ready to erupt again into painful, compelling consciousness.

I thought to settle, to be done with the mountain, to establish my sanctity on some little slope. But the mountain always shook me loose. A crack would open. A storm would come. Wrenched back to the current, pounded incessantly by water, by stones, I was forced to lose my latest grip, to slip ever lower down the side of the mountain. I was thrown against others' raw, rough edges. Resisting loudly, we clattered and cried. I seldom trusted or understood the work of the mountain, the painful plunges over jagged ledges down into boiling pools. Torn further and further from the glory at the summit, I despaired of the dream, being forced to let go.

Yet the mountain has never let go of me. I carry it with me. I am born of the mountain. I have been on the mountain the entire time. The mountain has never abandoned me. The mountain is in me, over me, around me. There is more to a mountain than its highest peak. We are all the mountain. I grasp the mountain and the mountain shakes me loose. I let go of the mountain and the mountain carries me. It molds me and shapes me and delivers me smooth at the end of the journey.

I am worn down. Here at the foot of the mountain I rest. A child may pick me up in wonder, feel the mystery in her palm, press me smooth against her cheek, taste the mountain in me full against her lips; then toss me back, captivated by another stone or a frog or flower, dragonfly or fern.

Dappled sun, singing water, other stones touching me, other stones holding me, resting here together, supporting one another. The touch of fallen leaves floating by, the flick of minnows, the slime of snails, rotten roots we have clung to, they all pass by. The memory of a child's cheek, hand, kiss, release.

Kiss. Release.

I had thought to be the mountain. I tumbled down here. It is enough. Oh, it is more than enough.